Organ of the International Association of Gerontology (IAG)

Gerontology

International Journal of Experimental, Clinical and Behavioural Gerontology

Founded 1957 by F. Verzàr as 'Gerontologia',
merged 1975 with 'Gerontologia Clinica',
founded 1959 by E. Woodford-Williams and A.N. Exton-Smith

KARGER

Printed in Switzerland
on acid-free paper by
Reinhardt Druck, Basel

Appears bimonthly:
1 volume per year
(6 issues)

Gerontology

Guidelines for Authors

Gerontology publishes manuscripts on all aspects of experimental, clinical, and behavioural science research into the aging process. It accepts particularly high-quality, original research papers in all disciplines of gerontological research.

Gerontology welcomes those submissions which represent a conceptual advance or an original approach to the understanding of the molecular or behavioural basis of aging. From the clinical angle we would like papers of general interest submitted concerning the aetiology, pathogenesis, prevention and treatment of diseases or abnormalities of the elderly. Papers in the fields of neuroscience, cardiology, infectious disease and immunology, cancer, and epidemiology, to name just a few subjects of interest, will find a place in *Gerontology*, as will those reflecting current developments in the behavioural sciences.
In the section 'Reviews', themes of general interest including nutrition, longevity, psychology, demography, socioeconomic problems in old age such as health-care financing, benefits and risks of physical exercise, and normal and abnormal aging are welcome.

Studies on drugs, e.g. double-blind trials, are already covered by most of the other gerontology journals and are therefore *not considered* for publication in *Gerontology*.
Experimental papers dealing with *mechanisms of developmental phenomena* and which are not related to changes due to old age are not of interest for *Gerontology*.
Authors should indicate whether they wish their article to be considered for the Experimental, Clinical or Behavioural Science section. Manuscripts may be submitted in the following categories:

Review Articles
Original Research Papers/Experimental Section
Original Research Papers/Clinical Section
Original Research Papers/Behavioural Science Section
Debate
Short Communications
Letters to the Editor
Book Reviews
Announcements

Submission

Only original papers written in English are considered and should be sent to:

Prof. Dr. W. Meier-Ruge
Institut für Pathologie der Universität Basel
Gerontologische Forschung
Schönbeinstrasse 40
CH–4003 Basel (Switzerland)

Manuscripts from North America should be sent to:

Donald K. Ingram, PhD
National Institute on Aging
National Institutes on Health
Gerontology Research Center
5600 Nathan Shock Drive
Baltimore, MD 21224 (USA)

Tel. (410) 558 8180
Fax (410) 558 8323
E-Mail doni@vax.grc.nia.nih.gov

Only manuscripts that conform with the Guidelines for Authors will be considered.

Manuscripts should be submitted in triplicate (with three sets of illustrations of which one is an original), typewritten double-spaced on one side of the paper, with a wide margin.

***A statement signed by all authors* saying that they agree with the publication of the paper should accompany the manuscript.**

Original Research Papers must describe new research results, not published or under consideration in another journal. Note: **A maximum of *six authors* is allowed.** All papers should be arranged with an Introduction, Methods, Results and Discussion. An exception is made for Reviews and Debate articles. Abbreviations should be explained and limited to a minimum. All terms abbreviated in the text, abstract and in the figures must, on the first occasion, be given in full, followed by the abbreviation (e.g. electrocardiogram (ECG)). Any papers dealing, partly or wholly, with basic science should include a few lines of description to any concept which may not be well known to some readers who are primarily practising clinicians.

Critical Reviews are either invited by the Editors, or may be submitted for consideration. Invited reviews, if accepted, are not subject to page charges.

The *Debate* Section publishes arguments, critical statements and theoretical papers reflecting the authors' views on mechanisms of the aging process at all levels of biological and medical organization and clinical matters of general interest and controversy.

The *Short Communications* Section is reserved mainly for case reports. Short Communications may be limited to two printed pages.

Letters addressed to the Editor are encouraged if they directly concern articles previously published in this journal and clinical subjects related to the matters discussed. The editor reserves the right to submit copies of such letters to the authors of the articles concerned prior to publication in order to permit them to respond in the same issue of the journal. But letters on general scientific or medical subjects in gerontology are also welcome. Letters to the Editor should be no longer than one printed page.

Disk submission

Do not send a disk before the paper is accepted for publication. The accepted manuscript must match the file on disk exactly. For details, refer to 'Disk Submission' or www.karger.com/journals/disksub.htm. Copy-editing will be executed from the disk version of your manuscript.

Conditions

All manuscripts are subject to editorial review. Manuscripts are received with the explicit understanding that they are not under simultaneous consideration by any other publication or have not already been published. Submission of an article for publication implies the transfer of the copyright from the author to the publisher upon acceptance. Accepted papers become the permanent property of *Gerontology* and may not be reproduced by any means, in whole or in part, without the written consent of the publisher. It is the author's responsibility to obtain permission to reproduce illustrations, tables, etc. from other publications.

Arrangement

Title page: The first page of each paper should indicate the title, the authors' names, the institute where the work was conducted, and a short title for use as running head.

Full address: The exact postal address of the corresponding author complete with postal code must be given at the bottom of the title page. Please also supply phone and fax numbers, as well as e-mail address.

Key words: For indexing purposes, a list of 3–7 key words (no abbreviations) in English is needed.

Each *Abstract* should be structured as follows:

Background: What prompted the study?
Objective: What is the purpose of the study?
Methods: How was the study carried out?
Results: What are the most important findings?
Conclusion: What is the most important conclusion?

The abstract should not exceed 350 words, and any abbreviations must be explained.

Footnotes: Avoid footnotes. When essential, they are numbered consecutively and typed at the foot of the appropriate page.

Tables and illustrations: Tables and illustrations (both numbered in Arabic numerals) should be prepared on separate sheets. Tables require a heading and figure legends should be supplied on a separate sheet. For the reproduction of illustrations, only good drawings and original photographs will be accepted; negatives or photocopies cannot be used. Due to technical reasons, figures with a screen background should not be submitted. When possible, group several illustrations on one block for reproduction (max. size 180 × 223 mm) or provide crop marks. On the back of each illustration, indicate its number, the author's name, and 'top' with a soft pencil. Electronically submitted b/w half-tone and color illustrations must have a final resolution of 300 dpi after scaling, line drawings one of 800–1200 dpi.

Color illustrations: Up to 6 color illustrations per page can be integrated within the text at the special price of CHF 660.–/USD 545.00 per page. Color illustrations are reproduced at the author's expense.

KARGER

Fax +41 61 306 12 34
E-Mail karger@karger.ch
www.karger.com

The Guidelines for Authors are available at:
www.karger.com/ger_Guidelines

References: Identify references in the text with Arabic numerals [in square brackets]. Material submitted for publication but not yet accepted should be noted as 'unpublished data' and not be included in the reference list. The list of references should include only those publications cited in the text. Do not alphabetize; number references in the order in which they are first mentioned in the text. The surnames of the authors followed by initials should be given. There should be no punctuation other than a comma to separate the authors. Preferably, please cite all authors. Abbreviate journal names according to the Index Medicus system. (Also see International Committee of Medical Journal Editors: Uniform requirements for manuscripts submitted to biomedical journals. N Engl J Med 1997;336:309–315.)

Digital Object Identifier (DOI)
S. Karger Publishers supports DOIs as unique identifiers for articles. A DOI number will be printed on the title page of each article. DOIs can be useful in the future for identifying and citing articles published online without volume or issue information. More information can be found at www.doi.org.

Examples
(a) Papers published in periodicals: Sun J, Koto H, Chung KF: Interaction of ozone and allergen challenges on bronchial responsiveness and inflammation in sensitised guinea pigs. Int Arch Allergy Immunol 1997;112:191–195.
(b) Papers published only with DOI numbers: Theoharides TC, Boucher W, Spear K: Serum interleukin-6 reflects disease severity and osteoporosis in mastocytosis patients. Int Arch Allergy Immunol DOI: 10.1159/000063858.
(c) Monographs: Matthews DE, Farewell VT: Using and Understanding Medical Statistics, ed 3, revised. Basel, Karger, 1996.
(d) Edited books: Parren PWHI, Burton DR: Antibodies against HIV-1 from phage display libraries: Mapping of an immune response and progress towards antiviral immunotherapy; in Capra JD (ed): Antibody Engineering. Chem Immunol. Basel, Karger, 1997, vol 65, pp 18–56.

Page charges
There are no page charges for papers of up to 4 printed pages (i.e., 12 typewritten pages at 33 lines per page, 65 strokes per line, including tables, illustrations and references). Each additional complete or partial page is charged to the author at CHF 275.–/USD 196.00.

Galley proofs
Unless indicated otherwise, galley proofs are sent to the first-named author and should be returned with the least possible delay. Alterations made in galley proofs, other than the correction of printer's errors, are charged to the author. No page proofs are supplied.

Reprints
Order forms and a price list are sent with the galley proofs. Orders submitted after the issue is printed are subject to considerably higher prices.

Gerontology

General Information

Publication data: 'Gerontology' is published 6 times a year. Volume 50 with 6 issues appears in 2004.

Subscription rates: Subscriptions run for a full calendar year. Prices are given per year.
Personal subscription:

Print or Online	Print/Online combined
CHF 528.–	CHF 569.–
EUR 391.–	EUR 421.–
USD 422.50	USD 455.50
postage and handling	(added to print and print/online)
CHF 31.80 Europe,	CHF 47.10 Overseas
EUR 22.80	
USD 31.80	

Institutional subscription:

Print or Online	Print/Online combined
CHF 1056.–	CHF 1140.–
EUR 782.–	EUR 844.–
USD 845.00	USD 912.00
postage and handling	(added to print and print/online)
CHF 39.60 Europe,	CHF 58.80 Overseas
EUR 28.50	
USD 39.60	

Airmail surcharge: CHF 39.60 / USD 33.00
Discount subscription prices:
Int. Ass. of Gerontology; British Geriatric Society; Gerontological Soc.; American Geriatric Society.

Microforms: Please direct all enquiries and orders to:
University Microfilms Inc.
300 North Zeeb Road, P.O. Box 1346
Ann Arbor, MI 48106-1346 (USA)

Subscription orders: Orders can be placed at agencies, bookstores, directly with the Publisher
S. Karger AG, P.O. Box
CH–4009 Basel (Switzerland)
or with any of the following distributors:
Deutschland: S. Karger GmbH, Postfach
D–79095 Freiburg
France: Librairie Luginbühl
36, bd de Latour-Maubourg
F–75007 Paris
Great Britain, Ireland: S. Karger AG
4 Rickett Street
London SW6 1RU, UK
USA: S. Karger Publishers, Inc.
26 West Avon Road, P.O. Box 529
Farmington, CT 06085, USA
India, Bangladesh, Sri Lanka:
Panther Publishers Private Ltd.
33, First Main
Koramangala First Block
Bangalore 560 034, India
Japan: Karger Japan, Inc.
Yushima S Bld. 3F
4-2-3, Yushima, Bunkyo-ku
Tokyo 113-0034, Japan

Change of address: Both old and new address should be sent to the subscription source.

Single issues and back volumes: Information can be obtained through the Publisher.

Advertising: Correspondence and rate requests should be addressed to the Publisher.

Bibliographic indices: This journal is regularly listed in bibliographic services, including *Current Contents*® and Index Medicus/MEDLINE.

Fax +41 61 306 12 34
E-Mail karger@karger.ch
www.karger.com

The Journal Home Page is available at:
www.karger.com/ger

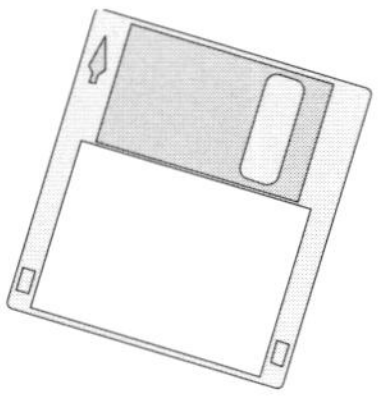

Disk Submission

A **comprehensive version** of these guidelines for the **submission of manuscripts and illustrations on disk** can be accessed online under **www.karger.com/disksubmission** or requested as a leaflet from the editorial department.

Please follow the general rules on style and arrangement in the **'Guidelines for Authors'** of the journal. Submit a **double-spaced printout** of your manuscript matching the file on disk exactly.

Technical Information
Store only data pertinent to this manuscript. Include your fonts (screen and printer fonts for Macintosh). For a **text only** manuscript, use a 3.5-inch disk. For **text and illustrations,** use 3.5 or 5.25 Magneto Optical Disc; CD-ROM (DOS or hybrid); iomega Zip/DOS (100 MB), or 44 MB, 88 MB or 200 MB SyQuest. Compress extensive data using ZIP format.

Data Description
Label your disk with the **title of the journal or book** for which it is submitted; a **short version** of the paper's title; your **name,** postal and e-mail address, fax and phone number; **hard- and software** used, including the version; and the **complete list of the file names.** File names consist of eight characters before the dot identifying the file and three characters after the dot identifying the application.

Text and Format
The **preferred word-processing package is MS-Word.** Other commonly used PC text programs and ASCII formats are accepted.
Update your data when you revise subsequent to the reviewer's or editor's decision and mark revisions clearly. Manuscripts accepted for publication are subject to **copy editing:** changes and/or questions will be marked in the manuscript, which will be returned to you with your disk and the galley proofs for checking.
Enter your text continuously flush left. Do not use any layout functions. Do not split words at the end of a line. **Do not use indentations.** Use a blank line before and a hard return at the end of paragraphs.
Arrange headings flush left. Insert only **one space after punctuation marks.** Insert Greek letters, mathematical symbols etc. with your word-processing program. Use **boldface and italics** as well as sub- and superscript where appropriate.
Tables are part of the text and should be placed at the end of the text file. Separate the individual parts of a table by lines. Use the tabulator instead of spaces. Format operation data on one line in the same column.

Legends to illustrations are part of the text and should also be listed at the end of the text file.

Illustrations
Store illustrations as separate files: do not integrate them in your text. Export **line drawings/vector graphics** as TIF, EPS or WMF format. Use Photoshop for processing and retouching **scanned half-tone images.** Save the original scan and the processed version. Export **black and white or color images** as TIF or EPS format in their anticipated size in print. **For detailed information** on how to submit illustration data on disk please consult the leaflet or **www.karger.com/disksubmission.**

KI 02 DISK

KARGER

Fax +41 61 306 12 34
E-Mail karger@karger.ch
www.karger.com

The Journal Home Page is available at:
www.karger.com/ger

Ignatius Nascher Prize of the City of Vienna in Geriatrics

The Ignatius Nascher Prize in Geriatrics will be awarded by the City of Vienna during next year's 7th Viennese International Geriatrics Conference.

The Sponsorship Prize (EUR 3630) will be awarded to applicants who have shown an important scientific contribution to the field of geriatrics, with a special emphasis on the areas of health promotion, prevention, diagnostics, therapeutics, rehabilitation or continued geriatric long-term care.

Closing date: 15 January 2004
Address: Prim. Dr. Katharina Pils
Ludwig Boltzmann Institute for
Interdisciplinary Rehabilitation in Geriatrics
SMZ-Sophienspital
Apollogasse 19
A–1070 Vienna (Austria)
E-Mail: ilse.howanietz@wienkav.at

Submission for Sponsorship Prize should include in triplicate:

1. the completed study including the project evaluation or the publication in a renowned scientific journal
2. an application letter
3. a curriculum vitae

The application may be presented by a person, a team or an institution. Former prize-awarded publications or theses submitted for the certificate of habilitation are excluded. The publication or completed and evaluated projects have to be presented in English or German. The summary should be structured according to the general publication rules, i.e. aim of the study, patients, material and methods; results; discussion; references; abstract.

The applicant must include a written statement, that all scientific participants were mentioned as co-authors or acknowledged.

The winner of the Sponsorship Prize will be informed by the end of March 2004, the prize-winning study should be presented during the 7th Viennese International Geriatrics Conference in May 2004.

Gerontology

Intraindividual Variability, Change, and Aging

Editors
Mary A. LUSZCZ, Adelaide
Mike MARTIN, Zurich
Scott M. HOFER, University Park, Pa.

3 figures and 6 tables, 2004

KARGER

Basel · Freiburg · Paris · London · New York ·
Bangalore · Bangkok · Singapore · Tokyo · Sydney

S. Karger
Medical and Scientific Publishers
Basel · Freiburg · Paris · London
New York · Bangalore · Bangkok
Singapore · Tokyo · Sydney

Drug Dosage
The authors and the publisher have exerted every effort to ensure that drug selection and dosage set forth in this text are in accord with current recommendations and practice at the time of publication. However, in view of ongoing research, changes in government regulations, and the constant flow of information relating to drug therapy and drug reactions, the reader is urged to check the package insert for each drug for any change in indications and dosage and for added warnings and precautions. This is particularly important when the recommended agent is a new and/or infrequently employed drug.

P.O. Box, CH–4009 Basel (Switzerland)
Printed in Switzerland on acid-free paper by
Reinhardt Druck, Basel
ISBN 3–8055–7684–6

KARGER

Fax + 41 61 306 12 34
E-Mail karger@karger.ch
www.karger.com

Vol. 50, No. 1, 2004

Gerontology

Contents

KARGER

Fax + 41 61 306 12 34
E-Mail karger@karger.ch
www.karger.com

Access to full text and tables of contents, including tentative ones for forthcoming issues: www.karger.com/ger_issues

Gerontology

Editorial

Gerontology 2004;50:5–6
DOI: 10.1159/000074381

What's It All about: Variation and Aging

Mary A. Luszcz

School of Psychology, Flinders University, Adelaide, Australia

Key Words
Cognitive aging · Intraindividual variability · Methodology

Those of us who arrived at the study of cognitive ageing following a traditional experimental approach have long searched for ways to understand the 'noise' in our data. This noise was a 'nuisance' that often arose from cross-sectional studies. Through them we crudely sought to understand ageing as a process, while relying on data derived from studies where age and cohort were inherently confounded and single observations were made at one point in time. To the extent that human development is all about intraindividual change, this approach was flawed, but reflected at least two beguiling assumptions.

One was that the confounding of age and cohort might not be so crucial in the study of such basic processes as cognition. Although Schaie and others [1] have shown repeatedly that this is not the case, still the experimentalist forged on. We also held to a belief that observation of age by condition interactions would show the way to what ageing was all about. What we didn't realize at the outset was that these interactions are exceptionally elusive. The 'hum' in the system partially contributed to this, but the way forward was not obvious. One thing that is clear in the series of papers that follows is that there is both a need, and many ways, to harness interindividual differences, intraindividual change and interindividual differences in intraindividual change to enable us to better understand ageing. The return of a more psychometric approach to understanding ageing has been in no small part a contributor to this methodological shift.

The content area of these papers derives mainly from cognitive and sensory ageing, but the lessons to be learned here are readily transferable to other domains. Is this emphasis because these constitute two of the areas most relevant to day-to-day functioning and quality of life? Perhaps it derives from our having developed exquisitely sensitive barometers to index cognition and the impact of sensory processes. Regardless, the challenge will be to (a) establish efficient as well as efficacious ways to undertake research that will not overtax our participants or our research resources and (b) extend these approaches to social and affective domains.

As a whole this series of papers raises important questions about how we conceptualize the ageing process. While the emphasis is on the statistical end of a theory-method continuum, the inseparability of these elements of analysis becomes obvious in each paper. The contributors develop theoretically-driven hypotheses about what could happen, given specific patterns of overall statistical relationships.

The core group of authors of these papers are part of a new generation of researchers of cognitive ageing who want to push the boundaries of evolving statistical techniques to re-visit old questions, e.g., of neural noise, fluid and crystallized intelligence and how gains at one point in time benefit later performance. They also emulate the

KARGER

Fax + 41 61 306 12 34
E-Mail karger@karger.ch
www.karger.com

0304–324X/04/0501–0005$21.00/0

Accessible online at:
www.karger.com/ger

Mary A. Luszcz
School of Psychology, Flinders University
GPO Box 2100
Adelaide 5001 (Australia)
Tel. +61 8 8201 2481, Fax +61 8 8201 3877, E-Mail mary.luszcz@flinders.edu.au

influence of the contextualism paradigm of the lifespan approach to human development [2].

Yet there is a paradox here, which is elegantly captured in the commentary by Nesselroade. He has a historical perspective that is sometimes overlooked by more junior colleagues with their sights set on the most recently downloaded manuscript. In my view, his strong message, and it is captured in these papers, is that it isn't the issues that are new, but rather the means that we have at our disposal to pursue them. In short, modern computers and computational algorithms that they can implement parsimoniously are part of that shift. Equally, if not more, important is the capacity of the researchers themselves to be part of a global village, easily able to communicate across great distances or at close range with relative frequency. In the pages that follow you will see some of the benefits of 'interactive minds' at work on questions that have vexed developmental psychologists since its beginnings.

References

1 Schaie KW: Adult intellectual development: The Seattle Longitudinal Study. New York, Cambridge University Press, 1996.

2 Baltes P, Smith J: New frontiers in the future of aging: From successful aging of the young old to the dilemmas of the fourth age. Gerontology 2003;49:123–135.

Gerontology

Gerontology 2004;50:7–11
DOI: 10.1159/000074382

Intraindividual Variability, Change, and Aging: Conceptual and Analytical Issues

Mike Martin[a] Scott M. Hofer[b]

[a]Department of Gerontopsychology, Institute of Psychology, Zurich, Switzerland; [b]Pennsylvania State University, University Park, Pa., USA

Key Words
Cognitive aging · Intraindividual variability · Longitudinal studies · Theories of aging · Adaptation

Abstract
Background: Developmental researchers use a variety of research designs to examine aging-related changes. Most longitudinal studies of aging are based on research designs that feature successive, widely spaced, assessments to estimate changes in cognitive performance. Such designs assume that short-term variations in cognitive performance are small relative to long-term changes or have modeled such phenomena as nuisance parameters. ***Objective:*** There is now sufficient empirical evidence to establish intraindividual cognitive variability as a systematic source of individual differences and of important predictive value for aging-relevant outcomes. ***Methods:*** After an overview of types of change, potential underlying processes, and adequate analytic designs, we discuss consequences for lifespan aging research. ***Results:*** We emphasize that interpretations of both cross-sectional and longitudinal results need to consider and specify theoretical assumptions about short-term and long-term changes. ***Conclusions:*** Above and beyond the analysis of long-term mean changes, short-term changes are an important aspect of aging-related change, and their analysis may help to explain psychological processes of adaptation.

Paper presented at the International Workshop on Methods Examining Variability in Lifespan Aging Research, Heidelberg, Germany, February 2002.

Research on aging examines ordered changes that can be meaningfully related to chronological age and age-graded periods of development across the lifespan. Theoretical positions differ widely with respect to the explanatory domain (e.g., emotions, intellectual performance, social behavior, or attitudes), the parts of the lifespan in focus (e.g., infants, children, adolescence, adulthood, or old age), the outcome variable in focus (e.g., well-being, health, intelligence, or professional success), the explanatory constructs (e.g., knowledge, inhibition, speed of processing), the length of time for developmental predictions (e.g., early childhood to old age vs. middle adulthood to old age), and the specificity of predictions. Overall, most theoretical positions and empirical findings speak to the question of long-term changes, i.e., how particular explanatory developmental parameters earlier in life influence the developmental outcome parameters such as well-being, health or intelligence later in life [1]. Hence, psychological aging research is generally focussing on the

KARGER
Fax + 41 61 306 12 34
E-Mail karger@karger.ch
www.karger.com

© 2004 S. Karger AG, Basel
0304–324X/04/0501–0007$21.00/0

Accessible online at:
www.karger.com/ger

Mike Martin
Institute of Psychology, Department of Gerontopsychology
Schaffhauserstrasse 15
CH–8006 Zürich (Switzerland)
Tel. +41 1 635 34 30, Fax +41 1 635 34 21, E-Mail m.martin@psychologie.unizh.ch

detection of reliable age-related long-term change in psychological processes such as thinking, learning, reasoning, emotions, personality, motivation, or, generally, behavior.

Most longitudinal studies of aging are based on research designs that feature successive, widely-spaced, assessments to estimate changes in cognitive performance. Such designs assume that short-term variations in cognitive performance are small relative to long-term changes. Indeed, if short-term temporal variability is moderate to high, then single assessments would likely produce imprecise estimates of an individual's characteristic level of cognitive functioning and has implications for estimates of individual change. Although the focus on long-term change has not emphasized short-term variation or has approached modeling such phenomena as nuisance parameters, short-term intraindividual variability has long been considered an interesting outcome in itself. There is now sufficient empirical evidence that establishes intraindividual cognitive variability as a substantial source of systematic performance variability between people, especially in older adults [2–5].

Of course, not all of the short-term intraindividual variability contains theoretically or practically meaningful information (see Nesselroade's commentary). In many cases, however, short-term intraindividual variability or change might contain meaningful information about psychological processes of interest. In fact, there may be many different manifestations of short-term change and several possible theoretical interpretations. For example, intraindividual short-term variability may be an early indicator of deficits [6] or later-onset declines [7]. With respect to the differentiation-dedifferentiation [8] or the 'common cause' hypothesis [9], intraindividual short-term variability might be indicative of the structure of aging-related changes. Intraindividual short-term variability could also indicate adaptive behavior to cope with a stressful event or the limitations that go along with physical ailments. As an example, an increase in short-term intraindividual variability in extreme old age is not necessarily maladaptive. To maintain low levels of variability in developmental outcomes such as well-being or health requires a high level of regulatory effort. If, however, individual energy levels are low [e.g., 10], it might be maladaptive to invest energy in the stability of a particular outcome variable. Given limited resources, such efforts might affect functioning in other life domains, e.g., social activities. Instead, setting wider margins between a maximum and minimum value for the variability of a particular outcome variable may reduce the effort required to balance functioning in both domains. As a consequence, within- and across-domain short-term intraindividual variability might increase.

Theoretical Basis for Short-Term Intraindividual Variability

Theories of development that attempt to explain age-related changes should consider specifications of which short- and long-term intraindividual change relations are theory-relevant and to which time scales predictions apply. In addition to specifying that there should be age-related changes in both explanatory concepts (e.g., in speed) and aging-related outcomes (e.g., fluid intelligence), it is possible to specify what longitudinal short- and long-term relations are to be expected or if the theory even applies to particular time frames of change. As a consequence, to test the 'common cause' hypothesis, one may ask if independent dimensions of intellectual functioning are more highly related at extreme old ages compared to middle age, i.e., a long-term prediction, and/or if within persons of different ages there is an increase in the covariance of short-term fluctuations in performance in independent dimensions of intellectual functioning, i.e., a short-term prediction. In this context, hypotheses about within-person changes need to be formulated and tested separately from hypotheses about population mean changes [e.g., 11].

So far, there is little research on systematic intraindividual aging-related short-term variability, i.e., on the interaction between short-term intraindividual variability of explanatory parameters and intraindividual changes in other short-term developmental outcome parameters [e.g., 2–5]. There is also very little research on the predictive value of short-term intraindividual variability on later short-term variability, long-term changes, or long-term outcomes [13]. With adequate research designs, the examination of short-term intraindividual variability offers new possibilities for developmental research in many domains of psychological functioning. Results from these study designs may help to answer questions about the generality vs. specificity of intraindividual variability and about age-related differences in the range of observable intraindividual short-term variability. In the long run, these designs might add to the specificity of theories and predictions and support the development of tools allowing the early detection of problematic development.

Conceptual Basis for Short-Term Intraindividual Variability

Conceptually, the aging of an individual can be considered the development of a dynamic system of functional and goal processes within the context of environmental and developmental tasks. The processes within the system can be described by four related concepts: The concept of homeostasis emphasizes steady state and optimal set points. Allostasis refers to the maintenance of stability through change. It emphasizes optimal operating ranges of physiological systems given cumulative effects of stress on health and longevity. The concept of allostatic load assumes that stability through change represents the cumulative, multi-system view of physiological toll that may be exacted on the body through attempts at adaptation. Rheostasis refers to the regulated, controlled change in set points. More specifically, to examine covariations between short-term changes, a number of processes potentially causing intraindividual changes over time can be assumed to occur: (a) calibrating processes to match behavioral responses to environmental demands [14]; (b) compensating processes to stabilize a particular goal function such as well-being [15]; (c) reactive processes after reaching a critical threshold value in one or more relevant domains [16]; (d) optimization processes to coordinate parallel processes aiming at stabilizing different goal functions or hierarchies of goal functions [17]; (e) processes of fitting strategies with environmental demand, e.g., when practice effects lead to frequent use of a single strategy [18]; (f) anticipatory processes to prepare reactions to potential environmental changes [19]; (g) search processes trying out different ways to adapt to changing environmental conditions [20], and (h) adaptive processes after resetting minimum and/or maximum threshold values for one or more goal functions due to lack of energy to compensate the impact of events or stress [21].

Research Designs to Examine Short-Term Intraindividual Variability

Age-related increases in intraindividual variability have often been ascribed to the lack of instrument reliability (and validity) that can only be overcome by the power of large samples. One other way of approaching short-term intraindividual variability is to control non-informative short-term fluctuations and to test for additional, statistically reliable short-term intraindividual variability that is theoretically and practically meaningful. The research designs in combination with the statistical methods described in the papers of this special section may thus take into account interindividual differences in intraindividual change within a number of developmental domains. More importantly, these approaches permit formulation and empirical tests of hypotheses about the processes influencing development and aging at the individual level of analysis.

One may, for example, assume that lower levels of intraindividual variability (i.e., stability) in important goal functions such as health, well-being or information processing performance, require (compensatory) energy [e.g., 10]. This assumption can only be examined with a focus on short-term intraindividual variability. From this perspective, lower levels of intraindividual short-term variability are adaptive when tasks require high precision, when persons are close to their maximum performance level (variability would mean a decrease), when the behavior shown is efficient, when sufficient resources are available to compensate for distractions, and when the person tries to maximize a single process or goal function (e.g., intellectual functioning). In the same case, higher levels of intraindividual short-term variability are adaptive when the optimal behavior is unknown and it is preferable to try the effectiveness of the available behaviors, when persons are close to the minimum of their performance level, when low levels of energy are available to compensate distractions, and when the focus is on the optimization of two or more processes or goal functions (e.g., intellectual functioning and social activities). Across the lifespan, the precision required by tasks encountered, the availability of effective strategies, the level of competence and energy, and the focus on one or more goal functions probably changes. Only if changes in short-term intraindividual variability are included in building or reformulating lifespan developmental theories do we have the chance to receive a more complete picture of the adaptive capacities of persons at different ages.

Sampling Time

The study of intraindividual variation and covariation is not new. The well-known short form of Cattell's [22] data box provides an analytical framework for sampling across time, variables, and participants, the long form of the data box included other important aspects for understanding individual development by examining the environmental background and phase of the background, state of the organism, and other static and time-varying aspects of the context and participant. Given the interest in intraindividual variation, decisions regarding the sampling of time within individuals requires attention. Traditionally, the importance of sampling time has not been emphasized in developmental and aging research. We do expect, however, that change over time can follow many forms and these are likely to be different for combinations of different people, outcomes, and age periods. In terms of aging research, change can be gradual for periods of midlife, abrupt and nonlinear if related to acute illness, and may rebound to the previous level and so be described as interrupted plateaus or transitional in nature [23]. If our focus is on individual-level processes, research designs must be sensitive to all types of change in order to identify patterns and magnitudes of change within individuals. Given both systematic and stochastic sources of fluctuation in individual characteristics over short periods of time, such designs must also be sensitive to intraindividual variation [24, 25].

The sampling of time will influence analysis and interpretation of intraindividual variability and short-term change. Indeed, we might expect that different intervals will yield different patterns of variability and result from different influences on the 'system' or individual. For example, we might consider sampling moment to moment (attentional lapses); within-test (fatigue, practice); within-session (fatigue, order effects, motivation); within day (time of day effects); across days or weeks (environmental perturbations, physical health, practice); months or years (characteristic change trajectory). There is an increasing interest and development of methods for the evaluation of temporal dynamics of these types [26, 27].

Temporal sampling designs can take many forms. One such design, the measurement burst design [28, 29], utilizes intensive measurements over a short period in time and follow-up with further measurement burst sessions after longer intervals and permits a window on individual-level characteristics as well as long-term change. Obtaining multiple, closely spaced assessments at each wave allows local temporal smoothing of data for each individual by averaging across multiple assessments. The addition of multiple indicators at each assessment permits further improvements in the modeling of random error components in models that incorporate true change. By improving measurement precision through multiple assessments or multiple indicators, such designs will increase statistical power to detect cognitive change at both the individual and aggregate sample levels and permit greater understanding of intraindividual processes within and across different time intervals. Indeed, measurement burst designs incorporating multiple indicators would permit an optimal opportunity for evaluating systematic short-term fluctuation and change. A further consideration is the context in which measurements are obtained. Most temporal sampling designs are performed under random contextual backgrounds, but individual variation in performance can be evaluated against defined contexts as well – more akin to experimental paradigms (e.g., levels of stress, dual-processing tasks).

Special Section on Intraindividual Variability

The set of manuscripts in this special section is based on presentations given at a conference on intraindividual variability held at The German Centre for Research on Ageing at The University of Heidelberg, February 2002. They represent a broad array of research that treats intraindividual variability and short-term change as important characteristics of an aging organism. The papers discuss issues of theory, domain specificity of changes, and state-of-the-art methodology. We see this renewed interest in intraindividual variation and short-term change as an important contribution to the study of aging. Intraindividual variability has often been dealt with as a confound or nuisance factor in single-measurement designs and repeated single-measurement designs. New applications of measuring intensive longitudinal designs, however, permit analysis of aggregate or characteristic level of functioning of the individual as well as features of variation and covariation within individuals. A commentary by John Nesselroade, a strong and consistent voice on the importance of studying intraindividual variation and covariation, concludes this special section.

References

1 Martin P, Martin M: Proximal and distal influences on development: Introducing the model of developmental adaptation. Dev Rev 2002;22:78–96.

2 Hultsch D, Hertzog C, Small BJ, McDonald-Miszczak L, Dixon RA: Short-term longitudinal change in cognitive performance in later life. Psychol Aging 1992;7:571–584.

3 Li S, Aggen SH, Nesselroade JR, Baltes PB: Short-term fluctuations in elderly people's sensorimotor functioning predict text and spatial memory performance: The MacArthur Successful Aging Studies. Gerontology 2001;47:100–116.

4 Nesselroade JR: Intraindividual variability in development within and between individuals. Eur Psychol 2001;6:187–193.

5 Strauss E, MacDonald SW, Hunter M, Moll A, Hultsch DF: Intraindividual variability in cognitive performance in three groups of older adults: Cross-domain links to physical status and self-perceived affect and beliefs. J Int Neuropsychol Soc 2002;8:893–906.

6 Schaie KW: The impact of longitudinal studies on understanding development from young adulthood to old age. Int J Behav Dev 2000;24:257–266.

7 Rowe JW, Kahn RL: Successful aging. Gerontologist 1997;37:433–440.

8 Li SC: Connecting the many levels and facets of cognitive aging. Curr Direct Psychol Sci 2002;11:38–43.

9 Christensen H, Mackinnon AJ, Korten A: The 'common cause hypothesis' of cognitive aging: Evidence for not only a common factor but also specific associations of age with vision and grip strength in a cross-sectional analysis. Psychol Aging 2001;16:588–599.

10 Fairclough SH: Mental effort regulation and the functional impairment of the driver; in Hancock PA, Desmond PA (eds): Stress, Workload, and Fatigue: Human Factors in Transportation. Mahwah, Erlbaum, 2001, pp 479–502.

11 Zimprich D, Martin M: Can longitudinal changes in processing speed explain longitudinal age changes in fluid intelligence? Psychol Aging 2002;17:690–695.

12 Kim JE, Nesselroade JR: Relationships among social support, self-concept, and wellbeing of older adults: A study of process using dynamic factor models. Int J Behav Dev 2003;27:49–63.

13 Eizenman DR, Nesselroade JR, Featherman DL, Rowe JW: Intraindividual variability in perceived control in a older sample: The MacArthur successful aging studies. Psychol Aging 1997;12:489–502.

14 Ceci SJ, Baker JG, Bronfenbrenner U: Prospective remembering, temporal calibration, and context; in Gruneberg MM, Morris PE (eds): Practical Aspects of Memory: Current Research and Issues. 1. Memory in Everyday Life. Oxford, Wiley, 1988, pp 360–365.

15 Staudinger U, Freund A, Linden M: Self, personality, and life regulation: Facets of psychological resilience in old age; in Baltes PB, Mayer KU (eds): The Berlin Aging Study: Aging from 70 to 100. New York, Cambridge University Press, 1999, pp 302–328.

16 Perlesz A, Kinsella G, Crowe S: Impact of traumatic brain injury on the family: A critical review. Rehabil Psychol 1999;44:6–35.

17 Sherrod LR: Using the selection, optimization and compensation model to take us one step further in developmental research. Hum Dev 2001;44:51–54.

18 West RL: Compensatory strategies for age-associated memory impairment; in Baddeley AD, Wilson BA (eds): Handbook of Memory Disorders. Oxford, Wiley, 1995, pp 481–500.

19 Mailles S, Marine C, Cellier J: Anticipatory behavior in a simulated bus traffic control task; in De Keyser V, d'Ydewalle G (eds): Time and the Dynamic Control of Behavior. Kirkland, Hogrefe & Huber, 1998, pp 303–317.

20 Luszcz M, Hinton M: Domain- and task-specific beliefs about memory in adulthood: A microgenetic approach. Aust Psychol 1995;47:54–59.

21 Martin P, Long MV, Poon LW: Age changes and differences in personality traits and states of the old and very old. J Gerontol 2002;57B:P144–P152.

22 Cattell RB: The data box: Its ordering of total resources in terms of possible relational systems; in Nesselroade JR, Cattell RB (eds): Handbook of Multivariate Experimental Psychology, ed 2. Perspectives on Individual Differences. New York, Plenum Press, 1988, pp 69–130.

23 Birren JE, Schroots JF: History, concepts, and theory in the psychology of aging; in Birren JE, Schaie KW (eds): Handbook of the Psychology of Aging, ed 4. San Diego, Academic Press, 1996, pp 3–23.

24 Baltes PB, Nesselroade JR: The developmental analysis of individual differences on multiple measures; in Nesselroade JR, Reese HW (eds): Life-span developmental psychology: Methodological issues. Oxford, Academic Press, 1973.

25 Nesselroade JR: The warp and the woof of the developmental fabric; in Downs RM, Liben LS (eds): Visions of aesthetics, the environment & development: The legacy of Joachim F. Wohlwill. Hillsdale, Lawrence Erlbaum, 1991, pp 213–240.

26 Boker SM, Nesselroade JR: A method for modeling the intrinsic dynamics of intraindividual variability: Recovering the parameters of simulated oscillators in multi-wave panel data. Multivar Behav Res 2002;37:127–160.

27 Molenaar PC: A dynamic factor model for the analysis of multivariate time series. Psychometrika 1985;50:181–202.

28 Nesselroade JR: The warp and the woof of the developmental fabric; in Downs RM, Liben LS (eds): Visions of Aesthetics, the Environment & Development: The legacy of Joachim F. Wohlwill. Hillsdale, Lawrence Erlbaum, 1991, pp 213–240.

29 Nesselroade JR, Schmidt-McCollam KM: Putting the process in developmental processes. Int J Behav Dev 2000;24:295–300.

Gerontology

Gerontology 2004;50:12–16
DOI: 10.1159/000074383

Static and Dynamic Longitudinal Structural Analyses of Cognitive Changes in Old Age

Paolo Ghisletta[a,b,c] Ulman Lindenberger[d]

[a]Center for Interdisciplinary Gerontology and [b]Faculty of Psychology and Educational Sciences, University of Geneva, Geneva, and [c]Center for Life Course and Life Style Study, Universities of Lausanne and Geneva, Switzerland; [d]Department of Psychology, Saarland University, Saarbrücken, Germany

Key Words

Latent growth and multilevel models · Cognitive aging

Abstract

Background: Among the main data-analytical advances of recent decades are Latent Growth Models (LGM) and Multilevel Models (MLM) for the analysis of longitudinal data. ***Objective:*** We discuss the relative advantages and disadvantages of the two analytical methods and offer some practical guidelines concerning the choice between LGM and MLM based on (a) completeness and balance of the data, (b) theoretical functional form of change examined, (c) examination of the error structure, (d) theoretical relations among differential level effects and differential change effects, and (e) role of time-invariant covariates. ***Methods:*** To discuss LGM and MLM, we provide illustrations from applications to the Berlin Aging Study (BASE) and the Swiss Interdisciplinary Longitudinal Study on the Oldest Old (SWILSO-O). ***Results:*** As predicted by two-component theories of lifespan cognition, performance on a vocabulary test (indicator of broad crystallized intelligence) did not decline over time, while scores on a digit letter test (indicator of broad fluid intelligence) decreased over 6 years. Differential level effects were obtained on both variables, while average and differential change effects were obtained only for the digit letter test. In a second set of analyses, we tested the error-free effect that a broad fluid intelligence indicator exerted on the latent yearly change in a broad crystallized intelligence indicator, and vice versa. In both data sets we obtained strong evidence for a more reliable effect of the fluid indicator on the change in the crystallized indicator. This evidence provided support for the dedifferentiation hypothesis of cognitive abilities in very old age. ***Conclusions:*** New insights into cognitive aging phenomena can be gained with proper applications of LGM and MLM. We posit that the choice between LGM and MLM and their specification rests on theoretical and empirical motives to be defined a priori.

During recent decades, lifespan developmental psychologists have witnessed some progress from conceptual, theoretical, methodological, and data-analytical perspectives [1, 2]. Among newer statistical models are Latent Growth Models (LGM) and Multilevel Models (MLM) for the analysis of longitudinal data. In this paper we discuss some applications of analytical models to the study of cognitive aging. To elucidate the themes discussed, we provide two empirical examples from our research.

KARGER

Fax + 41 61 306 12 34
E-Mail karger@karger.ch
www.karger.com

0304–324X/04/0501–0012$21.00/0

Accessible online at:
www.karger.com/ger

Paolo Ghisletta
Center for Interdisciplinary Gerontology, University of Geneva
Route de Mon-Idée 59
CH–1226 Thônex (Switzerland)
Tel. +41 22 305 66 04, Fax +41 22 348 90 77, E-Mail paolo.ghisletta@cig.unige.ch

Table 1. Description of variables from the BASE and SWILSO-O longitudinal designs

Cognitive domain	BASE occasion of measurement							SWILSO-O occasion of measurement		
	IA_1	IP_1	IA_2	IA_3	IP_3	IA_4	IP_4	1	2	3
Broad Gf/mechanic	DL	DL, IP	DL	DL	DL, IP	DL	DL, IP	CO	CO	CO
Broad Gc/pragmatic	–	VO, SW	–	–	VO, SW	–	VO, SW	CA	CA	CA
Time in study, years	0.00	0.13	1.95	3.76	3.99	5.55	6.03	0.00	1.35	2.31
n	516	516	361	244	208	164	132	376	289	247

IA = Intake assessment; IP = intensive protocol; DL = digit letter; IP = identical pictures; VO = vocabulary; SW = spot-a-word; CO = cross out; CA = category.

Latent Growth Models and Multilevel Models

LGM appeared in developmental psychology less than two decades ago [3]. MLM (highly similar to random effect, mixed, and hierarchical models) applied to longitudinal analyses developed independently [4, 5]. Today, both methodologies are commonly applied in the field of cognitive aging [e.g., 6–8]. The similarities and differences of LGM and MLM, although documented in the literature [e.g., 9–12], are not always clear and the empirical researcher is sometimes left wondering when to prefer one approach over the other. In short, MLM may be favored over LGM when: (a) the data are highly incomplete and/or unbalanced; (b) the functional form of change can be represented by a common mathematical function (e.g., polynomial, logistic, exponential); (c) the error structure can be represented by a common matrix (e.g., Toeplitz, independent-diagonal, auto-regressive, unstructured); (d) the theory examined does not mandate relations other than covariances among change components of different variables (i.e., static condition), and (e) the time-invariant covariates act uniquely as predictors of differential level and change effects. LGM may be favored over MLM when: (a) the degree of data incompleteness and/or unbalance is limited; (b) the change function is to be represented by more complex mathematical formulations or is to be estimated by the data; (c) the error structure is of theoretical interest, requiring flexible modeling; (d) the relations among the variables' level and change components cannot be represented by covariances (e.g., dynamic condition), and (e) the time-invariant covariates assume theoretical roles other than predictors of differential level and change effects. These conditions, however, can be adjusted and at times overwritten given sufficient familiarity with the analytical method chosen and the software utilized for their implementation.

To illustrate the notions mentioned above, we discuss applications of LGM and MLM to the Berlin Aging Study (BASE) [13] and the Swiss Interdisciplinary Longitudinal Study on the Oldest Old (SWILSO-O) [14].

Description of Research Studies

BASE is a multidisciplinary study of aging combining psychology, sociology and social policy, internal medicine and geriatrics, and psychiatry. At its onset (in 1989) it consisted of 516 individuals randomly sampled from the city registry of Berlin, Germany, stratified by gender and age (six groups of 5 years each from age 70; mean age = 84.9 years, age range = 69.7–103.1 years) [cf. 15]. The study is now in its fifth wave, but only data of the first four occasions are presented here. The first, third, and fourth waves of data collection were preceded by an initial assessment, during which fewer variables were administered. The full longitudinal cognitive battery included eight variables. However, for simplicity and illustration purpose, we will limit the analyses presented here to two markers of perceptual speed (digit letter and identical pictures) and two markers of verbal knowledge (vocabulary and spot-a-word). The data unbalance is apparent from table 1. In particular, the digit letter test was assessed seven times, while the other selected cognitive variables were limited to three assessments.

SWILSO-O is an interdisciplinary study of aging involving sociology, social psychology, cognitive psychology, social medicine, and econometrics. Two age-parallel cohorts comprise the sample, the first begun in 1994 (now in its eighth wave), the second in 1999 (currently in its fourth wave). The cognitive tests illustrated here were included only in the latter cohort. At inception, the second cohort comprised 376 participants stratified by geographical region (191 in rural Valais, Switzerland, vs. 185 in urban Geneva, Switzerland). The mean age at time 1 was 81.9 years, the age range 79.5–84.5 years. In contrast to the BASE cognitive design, the SWILSO-O cognitive design, albeit less comprehensive in its research pursuits, is balanced. Because of the shorter duration and the different age composition of the sample, the dropout rate at the end of the periods considered is smaller for SWILSO-O than for BASE (34.31% dropout rate in 2.31 years for SWILSO-O versus 74.42% throughout 6.03 years for BASE).

Static Relations between Broad Gf/Mechanic and Broad Gc/Pragmatic Markers

In this first set of analyses we were mainly interested in relations among cognitive variables of different domains, as hypothesized by two component theories of lifespan cognition [e.g., 16]. In particular, we were interested in the relationships among markers of broad Gf/mechanic and broad Gc/pragmatic domains. For didactical reasons, we will illustrate this application only with the digit letter (assessed seven times) and the vocabulary (assessed three times) tests of BASE. Classical model of change would have required that the variables analyzed be balanced, that is to say assessed an equal number of times. This inevitably would have resulted in the loss of more than half of the digit letter assessments. More modern models can not only accommodate incomplete data (unavoidable in longitudinal aging studies), but also unbalanced data.

The theoretical motivation of the analyses could be addressed with covariance relations among the level and change components of each variable. Moreover, we limited ourselves to polynomial change, and were not substantively motivated to investigate the structure of the residual effects of change. Hence, we favored the MLM approach. We defined change as the passing of time in years since the beginning of the study (i.e., we applied the time in study temporal definition because theoretical motives did not favor a different temporal definition). To obtain unbiased estimates of person-level covariances we centered the data around each person's mean of time in study [cf. 17–19].

We first studied the change function of each variable in a univariate fashion. This implied two separate, unrelated MLM. For each variable we studied the existence (i.e., significant difference from 0) of the random effect of the intercept (analogous to the variance of the level factor in LGM), fixed linear effect of time (i.e., mean of the linear slope factor), the random linear effect of time (i.e., variance of the linear slope factor), and the 'level 2' covariance (i.e., covariance between level and linear slope factors over participants). For the digit letter variable, assessed up to seven times, we also tested for fixed and random quadratic effects of time (i.e., for the mean and the variance of a quadratic slope factor) and these were found not to be statistically significant.

The two cognitive variables displayed reliable fixed and random intercept effects, while only digit letter displayed both reliable fixed and random linear time effects. Hence, on average, the sample's performance varied around the intercept of both the digit letter and vocabulary tests. However, average and differential linear change were displayed only on the digit letter test. The sample's performance on the vocabulary test stayed constant during the period considered. This situation (variation around the intercept of both tests and only variation around the linear slope of digit letter) gave rise to a three by three 'level 2' covariance matrix, that is a covariance matrix about the participants' heterogeneity around the intercepts and linear slope components. The covariance matrix contained the information about how much the sample varied on the intercept of both tests, how much the sample varied with the respect to the change in digit letter, and about the covariations among these components. Statistical testing of this covariance matrix concluded that all six elements were different from zero. The level variance was 90.75 for digit letter and 74.73 for vocabulary, while the slope variance of digit letter was 0.78. The correlation between the levels of digit letter and vocabulary was 0.64. The level and slope of digit letter correlated 0.49, while the slope of digit letter correlated 0.28 with the level of vocabulary.

As predicted by two-component theories of lifespan cognition, the broad Gf/mechanic marker displayed negative age changes within the present longitudinal observation interval of up to 6 years, while the broad Gc/pragmatic markers (e.g., vocabulary) did not [cf. 7]. Furthermore, the positive manifold phenomenon usually observed in cross-sectional studies among different cognitive abilities was here observed in latent space as a high correlation between the levels of both markers. The application of MLM allowed for the estimation of longitudinal age gradients of the broad Gf/mechanic marker and for relations among its level and linear change components. The level performance on the vocabulary test is not only informative of the level performance of the digit letter test, but also of the linear change in the digit letter test. However, no statement about timing (i.e., possible longitudinal lead-lag relationships among the two cognitive tests) can be inferred by inspecting the static level 2 covariance matrix.

Dynamic Relations between Broad Gf/Mechanic and Broad Gc/Pragmatic Markers

The second set of analyses [see also 20] was concerned with the testing of the dedifferentiation hypothesis of cognitive abilities in very old age, according to which performance on cognitive abilities is more generalized and less specific for older individuals, probably due to biological changes occurring at the brain level [16, 21, see also 22]. An untested assumption of the dedifferentiation hypothesis is that the broad Gf/mechanic markers affect directly the negative changes of broad Gc/pragmatic markers in old age.

The phenomenon investigated is hypothesized to occur over chronological age, so the most sensible definition of time is in terms of chronological age. The theoretical paradigm can no longer be examined with correlational relations among variables' characteristics. Rather, a sort of a cross-lagged parameter capturing the unidirectional effect exerted by one variable on the change of the other variable is needed. We hence opted for a variation of LGM, called Dual Change Score Model (DCSM) [23, 24]. The DCSM builds upon an LGM by defining the change in the variable of interest as a composite of the latent slope component and the auto-proportion effect due to the previous measurement, free of unrelated variance. In a multivariate setting the DCSM additionally defines the direct and error-free proportionality effect of one variable onto the change in the other variables. If this effect is statistically reliable, we say that the variables analyzed are linked dynamically, because the total effect of one variable on the other will change in time. The dynamic links are assessed independently of differences in reliability among the variables analyzed [20, 25].

Broad Gf/mechanic abilities were marked with a composite of the digit letter and identical pictures tests in BASE and the cross-out test in SWILSO-O, while broad Gc/pragmatic abilities with a composite of the vocabulary and spot-a-word tests in BASE and with a category (fruit) test in SWILSO-O. In each example, the effect size of the directional effect from the broad Gf/mechanic marker to the broad Gc/pragmatic marker was compared to the effect size of the opposite directional effect, after accounting for the auto-proportionality effects. In the BASE application estimating the parameter from perceptual speed to the change in verbal knowledge represented a χ^2 decrease of 31 points for one degree of freedom, while the opposite parameter (from verbal knowledge to the change in perceptual speed) amounted to a χ^2 drop of 10 points. The effect size of the former parameter was hence much greater. Similarly, in the SWILSO-O application estimating the parameter from perceptual speed to change in category caused a reduction of 4 χ^2 points, while estimating that from category to change in perceptual speed reduced the χ^2 index minimally. This application provides an empirical validation based on longitudinal data of the dedifferentiation hypothesis of cognitive abilities in old and very old age, independently of the sample's age heterogeneity.

Discussion

LGM and MLM extended the repeated-measures (M)ANOVA model by focusing not only on mean trajectories, but also on variance expectations, allowing for the separation of change-related variance from residual (e.g., error, retest effects) variance. Moreover, within LGM and MLM the distinction between level and change is formalized, so that several hypotheses about change correlating with initial level can be addressed statistically. Advanced applications of LGM and MLM allow also the modeling of non-polynomial change functions and of the empirical 'optimal' change function [e.g., 8].

The DCSM is a particular structural equation model nesting and combining the LGM-MLM and the more classical auto-regressive Markov-type model. Indeed, the DCSM retains the appeals of the LGM-MLM approach and adds the estimation of the auto-proportionality parameter. In multivariate applications the DCSM becomes particularly interesting because it allows for the estimation of the dynamic effects among changing variables, after accounting for unrelated variance, differences in reliability, auto-proportionality effects, as well as for the effects of covariates.

Conclusions

Recent advances in data analytical strategies allow researchers to relax many atheoretical assumptions of the past. Nowadays theories and hypotheses of aging can be more adequately tested and sounder conclusions can be drawn. However, any statistical model is only useful if its theoretical motives are explicit and the match between the theoretical and the empirical levels is as satisfying as possible. LGM and MLM are but two analytical strategies available to ameliorate theory testing processes. While they are clearly not free from problems (e.g., assumptions of data missing at random, of ergodicity, and of sample homogeneity), LGM, MLM, related models of change, and, most of all, their appropriate applications can deepen our understanding of behavioral processes dear to life-span developmentalists and gerontologists alike.

References

1 Collins LM, Horn JL: Best methods for the analysis of change. Washington, American Psychological Association, 1991.
2 Collins LM, Sayer M: New methods for the analysis of change. Washington, American Psychological Association, 2001.
3 McArdle JJ: Latent growth within behavior genetic models. Behav Genet 1986;16:163–200.
4 Laird NM, Ware JH: Random-effects models for longitudinal data. Biometrics 1982;38:963–974.
5 Bryk AS, Raudenbush SW: Application of hierarchical linear models to assessing change. Psychol Bull 1987;101:147–158.
6 Hofer SM, Christensen H, Mackinnon AJ, Korten AE, Jorm AF, Henderson AS, Easteal S: Change in cognitive functioning associated with ApoE genotype in a community sample of older adults. Psychol Aging 2002;17:194–208.
7 Singer T, Verhaeghen P, Ghisletta P, Lindenberger U, Baltes PB: The fate of cognition in very old age: Six-year longitudinal findings in the Berlin Aging Study (BASE). Psychol Aging 2003;18:318–331.
8 Ghisletta P, McArdle JJ: Latent growth curve analyses of the development of height. Structural Equation Modeling 2001;8:531–555.
9 McArdle JJ, Hamagami F: Multilevel models from a multiple group structural equation perspective; in Marcoulides GA, Schumaker RE (eds): Advanced Structural Equation Modeling. Issues and Techniques. Mahwah, Lawrence Erlbaum, 1996, pp 89–124.
10 Chou C-P, Bentler PM, Pentz MA: Comparisons of two statistical approaches to study growth curves: The multilevel model and latent curve analysis. Structural Equation Modeling 1998;5:247–266.
11 MacCallum RC, Kim C, Malarkey WB, Kiecolt-Glaser JK: Studying multivariate change using multilevel models and latent curve models. Multivar Behav Res 1997;32:215–253.
12 Lindenberger U, Ghisletta P: Modeling longitudinal changes in old age: From covariance structures to dynamic systems; in Dixon RA, Bäckman L, Nilsson LG (eds): New Frontiers in Cognitive Aging. Oxford, Oxford University Press, in press.
13 Baltes PB, Mayer KU: The Berlin Aging Study: Aging from 70 to 100. New York, Cambridge University Press, 1999.
14 Lalive d'Epinay C, Pin S, Spini D: Présentation de SWILSO-O, une étude longitudinale suisse sur le grand âge: L'exemple de la dynamique de la santé fonctionnelle. Année Gérontol 2001; 15:78–96.
15 Lindenberger U, Gilberg RD, Little TD, Nuthmann R, Pötter U, Baltes PB: Sample selectivity and generalizability of the results of the Berlin Aging Study; in Baltes PB, Mayer KU (eds): The Berlin Aging Study: Aging from 70 to 100. New York, Cambridge University Press, 1999, pp 56–82.
16 Lindenberger U: Lifespan theories of cognitive development; in Smelser NJ, Baltes PB (eds): International encyclopedia of the social and behavioral sciences. Oxford, Elsevier, 2001, pp 8848–8854.
17 Wainer H: The centercept: An estimable and meaningful regression parameter. Psychol Sci 2000;11:434–436.
18 Kreft IGG, de Leeuw J, Aiken LS: The effect of different forms of centering in hierarchical linear models. Multivariate Behav Res 1995;30: 1–21.
19 Mehta PD, West SG: Putting the individual back into individual growth curves. Psychol Methods 2000;5:23–43.
20 Ghisletta P, Lindenberger U: Age-based structural dynamics between perceptual speed and knowledge in the Berlin Aging Study: Direct evidence for ability dedifferentiation in old age. Psychol Aging, in press.
21 Baltes PB, Lindenberger U, Staudinger UM: Life-span theory in developmental psychology; in Lerner RM (ed): Handbook of Child Psychology. 1. Theoretical Models of Human development. New York, Wiley, 1998, pp 1029–1143.
22 Li S-C, Lindenberger U, Hommel B, Aschersleben G, Prinz W, Baltes PB: Lifespan transformations in the couplings between intellectual abilities and constituent cognitive processes. Psychol Sci, in press.
23 McArdle JJ, Hamagami F: Latent difference score structural analyses for linear dynamic analyses with incomplete longitudinal data; in Collins LM, Sayer M (eds): New Methods for the Analysis of Change. Washington, American Psychological Association, 2001, pp 137–175.
24 Hamagami F, McArdle JJ: Advanced studies of individual differences linear dynamic models for longitudinal data analysis; in Marcoulides GA, Schumacker RE (eds): New Developments and Techniques in Structural Equation Modeling. Mahwah, Lawrence Erlbaum, 2001, pp 203–246.
25 McArdle JJ, Hamagami F, Meredith W, Bradway KP: Modeling the dynamic hypotheses of Gf-Gc theory using longitudinal life-span data. Learn Indiv Differ 2000;12:53–79.

Gerontology

Gerontology 2004;50:17–21
DOI: 10.1159/000074384

Short-Term versus Long-Term Longitudinal Changes in Processing Speed

Daniel Zimprich[a] Scott M. Hofer[b] Marja J. Aartsen[c]

[a]Department of Gerontopsychology, University of Zurich, Zurich, Switzerland; [b]Department of Human Development and Family Studies, Pennsylvania State University, University Park, Pa., USA; [c]Department of Sociology and Social Gerontology, Free University of Amsterdam, Amsterdam, The Netherlands

Key Words
Cognitive aging · Nested growth model · Learning · Practice

Abstract
Background: Previous longitudinal studies of cognitive aging have focused on long-term performance changes. A recent surge of research has demonstrated that there are reliable interindividual differences in short-term cognitive performance changes. ***Objective:*** The present study links these two pathways of cognitive aging research by examining the association between short-term (learning, practice) versus long-term (development) changes in processing speed. ***Methods:*** Data from 963 elderly participants come from the Longitudinal Aging Study Amsterdam (LASA). ***Results:*** Nested latent growth curve analyses show that the amount of learning or practice in processing speed at first measurement occasion is positively related ($r = 0.72$) to individual differences in development of processing speed across 6 years. ***Conclusions:*** Short-term learning or practice gains in processing speed are positively associated with long-term developmental changes in processing speed in the elderly.

People's cognitive performance may vary considerably, not only across months or years, i.e., long-term time periods, but also from moment-to-moment, hour-to-hour, day-to-day, i.e., across short-term time periods. Long-term cognitive changes in old age have been the focus of many longitudinal studies, which have demonstrated that, on average, a variety of cognitive abilities decline with aging, but that there are reliable interindividual differences in rates of intraindividual change [1–3]. Recently, researchers in the field of cognitive aging have identified that the amount of moment-to-moment or day-to-day performance changes in cognitive tasks might also be an indicator of reliable individual differences in old age [4–6]. Because short-term cognitive performance changes are not always functionally related to time in the sense of growth or decline, but rather represent performance 'oscillations' or 'fluctuations,' these studies have used intraindividual performance variability as an index of moment-to-moment or day-to-day cognitive changes.

An important extension of previous studies that examined either short-term or long-term cognitive performance changes consists of investigating the association between these two facets of cognitive change. That is, examining the relationship between cognitive changes based on different time scales, or between 'microdevelopment' and 'macrodevelopment' [7] of cognition in old age. An association between short-term and long-term cognitive performance changes would be extremely valuable

KARGER

Fax + 41 61 306 12 34
E-Mail karger@karger.ch
www.karger.com

0304–324X/04/0501–0017$21.00/0

Accessible online at:
www.karger.com/ger

Daniel Zimprich
Department of Gerontopsychology, University of Zürich
Schaffhauserstrasse 15
CH–8006 Zürich (Switzerland)
Tel. +41 1 635 3232, Fax +41 1 635 3221, E-Mail d.zimprich@psychologie.unizh.ch

from a theoretical point of view, because it would provide new insights into the dynamics of cognitive development in the elderly. Practically, if the association between micro- and macrodevelopment of cognition is substantive and reliable, it would be possible to predict long-term cognitive performance changes from short-term cognitive performance changes. Short-term cognitive performance changes might then, e.g., be used as a diagnostic tool for the early identification of dementia [8].

There are at least two alternative approaches in examining the relationship between micro- and macrodevelopment of cognition in old age. (1) Linking short-term cognitive performance oscillations or fluctuations, i.e., intraindividual variability, to long-term cognitive performance changes. Using this approach, one would investigate whether interindividual differences in the amount of short-term intraindividual variability are predictive of interindividual differences in the amount of long-term cognitive change. Modelling short-term changes would then require estimating random individual deviations from a fixed mean intraindividual variance, which, however, could render invalid statistical tests based on normality. (2) Linking short-term cognitive performance changes that are functionally related to time, e.g., learning or practice, to long-term cognitive performance changes. By means of this approach, one would examine if interindividual differences in the amount of intraindividual learning or practice are predictive of interindividual differences in long-term cognitive change. This second approach fits into the tradition of the 'testing-the-limits' method, which aims at explicating the role of learning within short time periods in long-term cognitive development [9].

Both approaches might be followed for one cognitive ability only or for different cognitive abilities simultaneously. If, for example, speed of information processing is considered a relevant explanatory variable for the decline in other cognitive abilities with advancing age [10], an important issue to examine empirically would be whether interindividual differences in short-term changes of processing speed are related to interindividual differences in long-term changes of other cognitive abilities. Thus, the association between short-term and long-term performance changes across different cognitive abilities may also be relevant for current theories of cognitive aging.

In the present study, we investigated the relationship between short-term, within-session learning or practice changes in processing speed across three trials and long-term changes in processing speed across three measurement occasions over 6 years. Statistical analyses of this data situation could, at first glance, rely on 'piecewise' growth models, which link growth rates during two (or more) different time periods [11]. However, piecewise growth models require change in two (or more) different periods be measured on the same time scale, e.g., days or years. For the data sampling scheme described above this does not seem warranted. Furthermore, piecewise growth models are designed to capture change processes that are measured across different points in time. Note, however, that the data at hand are 'nested', that is, within measurement occasions there are three processing speed trials.

It might thus seem more appropriate to view the data sampling scheme as a three level structure [12], with trials being nested within measurement occasions and measurement occasions being nested within persons. The argument would then be that trials within a measurement occasion are more strongly related to each other than are trials across measurement occasions. However, a three-level model describes only one nested growth process, whereas the aim of the present study is to examine different growth processes simultaneously, namely, three short-term growth processes within measurement occasions (learning, practice) and one long-term growth process across measurement occasions (development of processing speed).

Hence, in addressing the issue of short-term and long-term change processes, we nested within-measurement occasion latent growth models capturing learning and practice into an across-measurement occasion latent growth model that captures development of processing speed (fig. 1). We hypothesized that individual differences in learning and practice would be predictive of individual differences in the development of processing speed. More specifically, we expected that participants showing more learning and practice at first measurement occasion would show less decline in processing speed across the three measurement occasions due to greater cognitive plasticity [13, 14].

Method

Sample

Data come from the Longitudinal Aging Study Amsterdam (LASA) [15]. Details regarding the sampling scheme of LASA, the measurement protocol, the complete sample, and longitudinal attrition are reported elsewhere [16]. Participants with complete data (n = 963) on three measurement occasions (T1: 1992/93; T2: 1995/96; T3: 1998/99) were included in the present study. Mean age at the first measurement occasion (1992/1993) was 71.08 years (SD = 6.12, 61–85 years), 50% of the sample were female.

Measures

Processing Speed. Speed of information processing was measured using a modified version of the Alphabet Coding Task [17]. A work-

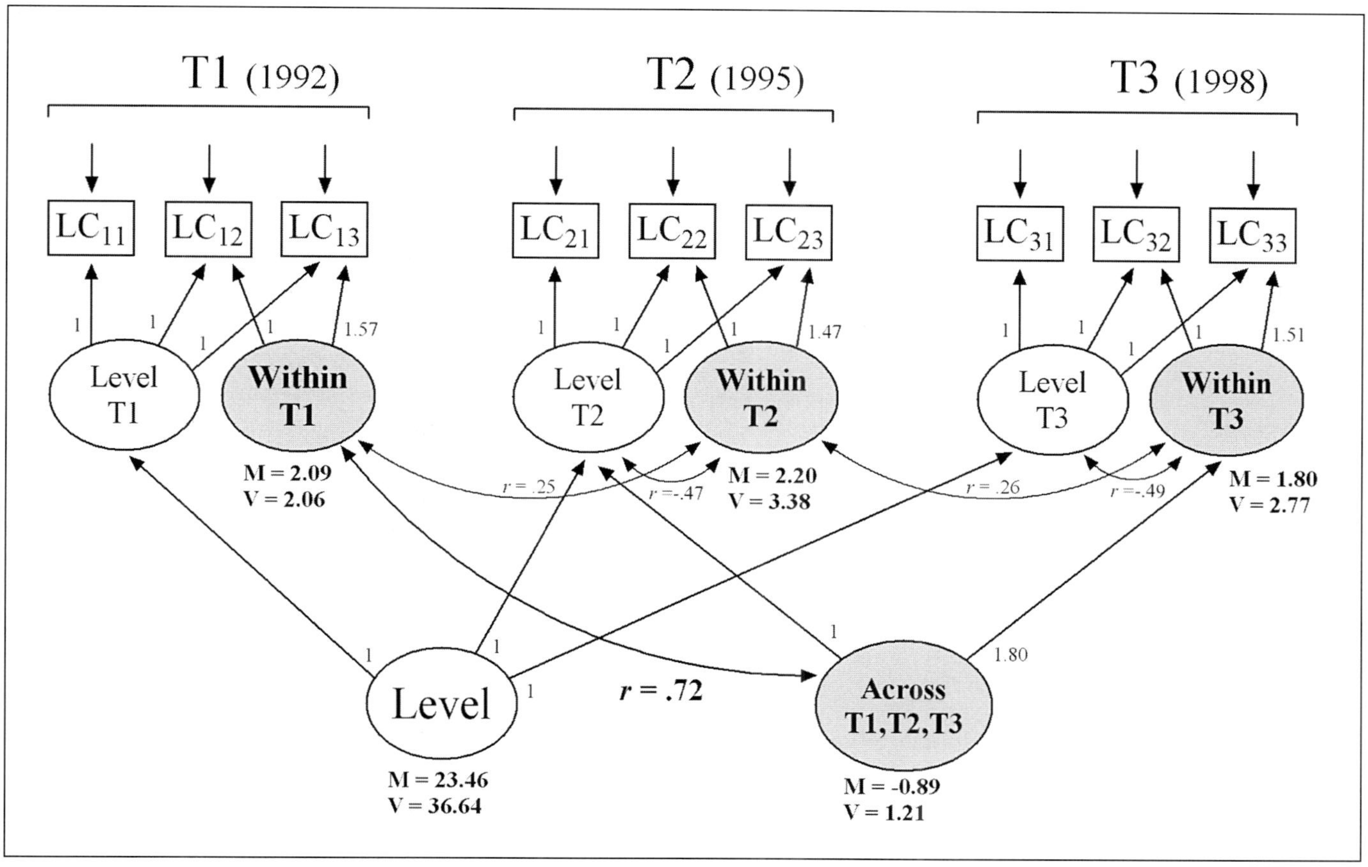

Fig. 1. Within- and across-measurement occasion latent growth model of processing speed. n = 963; χ^2 = 39.8; d.f. = 23; p < 0.02; CFI = 1.00; RMSEA = 0.028; LC = Letter Coding Task; M = mean; V = variance.

ing sheet with a Letter-Letter code table and several rows of characters with blanks underneath was presented to the participants. Participants were instructed to name as quickly and accurately as possible the characters that, according to the code table, should be used to fill up the blanks underneath the printed characters. This procedure was repeated in three trials of one minute each. The score for each trial of the Letter Coding Task consisted of the number of correctly completed combinations. Thus, at each measurement occasion there were three measures of processing speed, namely, the three trials of the Letter Coding Task.

Modelling Description

Let y_{ijk} represent the result of the Letter Coding Task of person i at measurement occasion j and within-measurement occasion trial k. A Level 1 linear growth model of within-measurement occasion changes at measurement occasion j would then be

$$y_{ijk} = \beta_{ij0} + \beta_{ij1}x + e_{ijk},$$

where β_{ij0} is the result of the first trial of person I at measurement occasion j, β_{ij1} is the amount of linear growth of person i in the second and third trial compared to the first trial, x represents the number of the trial minus 1, and e_{ijk} is a residual. Interindividual differences in β_{ij0} and β_{ij1} are modelled at Level 2, i.e., the person-level within-measurement occasion model:

$$\beta_{ij0} = \beta_{0j0} + r_{ij0},$$

$$\beta_{ij1} = \beta_{0j1} + r_{ij1},$$

where β_{0j0} is the mean result of the first trial of the Letter Coding Task across persons at the jth measurement occasion, β_{1j1} is the mean linear across-trial growth of the Letter Coding Task across persons at the jth measurement occasion, and r_{ij0} and r_{ij1} represent random effects (with zero means), i.e., interindividual differences.

Compared to standard linear growth models, there is a second Level 1 and a second Level 2 model that capture across-measurement occasion linear growth. Here, one has to decide which growth is to be modelled: Across-measurement occasion growth in the first within-measurement occasion trial, i.e. y_{i11}, y_{i21}, and y_{i31}, the second within-measurement occasion trial y_{i12}, y_{i22}, y_{i32}, or the third within-measurement occasion trial y_{i13}, y_{i23}, y_{i33}. We chose to model across-measurement occasion growth in the first trial of the Letter Coding Task, which may be considered development in processing speed. As an alternative, one could model growth in the third trial of the Letter Coding Task, which might be seen as development in the reserve capacity of processing speed. A Level 1 linear growth model of across-measurement occasion changes would then read

$$\beta_{ij0} = \beta_{i00} + \beta_{i10}t + e_{ij0},$$

where β_{ij0} is the result of the first trial of person i at measurement occasion j, β_{i00} is the result of the first trial of person i at the first measurement occasion, β_{i10} is the amount of linear growth of person i in the first trial at the second and third measurement occasion, t represents the number of years elapsed since the first measurement occasion, and e_{ij0} is a residual. Interindividual differences in β_{i00} and β_{i10} are modelled as:

$$\beta_{i00} = \beta_{000} + r_{i00},$$

$$\beta_{i10} = \beta_{010} + r_{i10},$$

where β_{000} is the mean result of the first trial of the Letter Coding Task across persons at the first measurement occasion, β_{010} is the mean linear growth of the first trial of the Letter Coding Task across persons and across measurement occasions, and r_{i00} and r_{i10} represent random effects (with zero means).

Thus, the complete growth model of within- and across-measurement occasion changes is:

$$y_{ijk} = \beta_{i00} + \beta_{i10}t + e_{ij0} + \beta_{ij1}x + e_{ijk}.$$

In total, there are 5 five random variances: (1) Initial status in the first trial at the first measurement occasion, (2) across-trial growth at the first measurement occasion, (3) across-trial growth at the second measurement occasion, (4) across-trial growth at the third measurement occasion, and (5) across-measurement occasion growth in the first trial (fig. 1).

In order to address the issue of an association between short-term and long-term changes in processing speed, the covariances between the respective random effects can be modelled. If, for example, the covariance between the random effect of within-measurement occasion growth at the first measurement occasion and the random effect of across-measurement occasion growth is statistically significant and positive, this would imply that short-term learning or practice in processing speed are predictive of long-term development in processing speed. All analyses were conducted using *Mx* [18].

Results

Figure 1 depicts the accepted latent growth curve model of within-and across-measurement occasion changes in processing speed. Results may be summarized as follows. (1) Within the first measurement occasion (T1: 1992/93), growth is nonlinear: Between the first and the second trial of the Letter Coding Task, there is an average performance increase of 2.09 points, whereas between the first and the third trial there is an average performance increase of 1.57 × 2.09 = 3.28 points. Analogous nonlinear growth is present within the second and the third measurement occasion. (2) Across the three measurement occasions, there is a non-linear performance decline in the first trial: Starting with an average Letter Coding performance of 23.46 points in the first trial at the first measurement occasion, at the second measurement occasion average performance is 23.46 – 0.89 = 22.57, and at the third measurement occasion average performance is 23.46 – (1.80 × 0.89) = 21.86. (3) Both for the within-measurement occasions growth and the across-measurement occasions growth there are reliable interindividual differences in the amount of growth, as is indicated by the statistically significant variances of the slope factors. (4) Within-measurement occasion growth at T1 is positively related to within-measurement occasion growth at T2 (r = 0.25), implying that those improving their performance more within T1 tend to also increase their performance more within T2. (5) Within-measurement occasion growth at T2 is positively associated with growth at T3 (r = 0.26), which implies that those improving their performance more within T2 tend to also increase their performance more within T3. (6) First trial performance at T2 is negatively related to growth at T2 (r = –0.47). That is, at T2, those with a higher performance at the first trial improve their performance across trials less than those with a lower performance. (7) First trial performance at T3 is negatively related to growth at T3 (r = –0.49). Hence, those with a lower performance at the first trial improve their performance across trials more than those with a higher performance. (8) The fit of the accepted model is excellent (χ^2 = 39.8, d.f. = 23, $p < 0.02$; CFI = 1.00, RMSEA = 0.028). A power analysis revealed that statistical power against 'true' RMSEA values of 0.08 and 0.05 was 1.00 and 0.88, respectively, which provides further support for an excellent model fit [19].

Of special interest are the relations between within-measurement occasion growth and across-measurement occasion growth. Only one out of three possible relations reached statistical significance, namely, the covariance between within-measurement occasion growth at T1 and the across-measurement occasion growth (1.144, SE 0.271), which corresponds to a correlation of r = 0.72 (90% confidence interval: 0.48–0.95). In order to validate this result, we used a bootstrap resampling approach comprising 1,000 bootstrap samples of size 963 [20]. Bootstrap analyses indicated that bias in the covariance between within-measurement occasion growth at T1 and the across-measurement occasion growth was minimal (–0.020), which suggests that the point estimate is relatively stable.

Thus, interindividual differences in the amount of growth within T1 account for 52% (23–90%) of interindividual differences in the amount of growth across measurement occasions. This finding implies that interindividual differences in the amount of learning or practice across the three trials of the Letter Coding task in 1992/93, i.e., short-term changes in processing speed at first measurement occasion, are highly predictive of individual differences in the development of processing speed, i.e., long-term changes within 6 years. According to this result, then, learning or practice within short time periods is positively associated with long-term cognitive development.

Discussion

The main finding of this study is that short-term processing speed changes are related to long-term processing changes. More specifically, individual differences in learning or practice gains across three trials of a Letter Coding task at first measurement occasion correlate 0.72 with individual differences in Letter Coding performance changes across the three measurement occasions. Short-term processing speed changes are thus highly predictive of long-term processing speed development in old age. If one considers the three trials of the Letter Coding task as a shortened variant of 'testing-the-limits' [9], the amount of reserve capacity in processing speed may predict future development in processing speed. However, before drawing final conclusions, a replication of our main finding involving a larger number of trials and measurement occasions seems warranted.

A potential limitation of this study is that we have chosen to include only participants with complete data records. More detailed analyses should use all available data by including participants with incomplete data as well, which may lead to less biased parameter estimates. Moreover, because the sample is inherently cross-sectional, it seems reasonable to incorporate age as a predictor of changes or to set up different latent growth curve models for different age groups. Finally, standard latent growth models rely on the assumption that individual change processes are of the same functional form, e.g., linear, for all persons. Using latent growth mixture modelling, however, it would be possible to discriminate between different sub-populations that, should they exist, show different patterns of change.

Still, our results suggest that short-term learning or practice gains have something in common with long-term developmental processes of cognition in the elderly. If true, then short-term learning or practice gains might be used as a diagnostic tool to identify persons with a high risk of cognitive decline. This, of course, would require more than the three trials of a cognitive task in order to get more precise estimates of short-term learning or practice gains.

References

1 Hultsch DF, Hertzog C, Dixon RA, Small BJ: Memory Change in the Aged. Cambridge, Cambridge University Press, 1998.
2 Sliwinski MJ, Buschke H: Cross-sectional and longitudinal relationships among age, cognition, and processing speed. Psychol Aging 1999;14:18–33.
3 Zimprich D, Martin M: Can longitudinal changes in processing speed explain longitudinal age changes in fluid intelligence? Psychol Aging 2002;17:690–695.
4 Hultsch DF, MacDonald SWS, Dixon RA: Variability in reaction time performance of younger and older adults. J Gerontol B Psychol Sci Soc Sci 2002;57B:P101–P115.
5 Rabbitt P, Osman P, Moore B, Stollery B: There are stable individual differences in performance variability, both from moment to moment and from day to day. Q J Exp Psychol A 2000;54A:981–1003.
6 West R, Murphy KJ, Armilio ML, Craik FIM, Stuss DT: Lapses of intention and performance variability reveal age-related increases in fluctuations of executive control. Brain Cogn 2002; 49:402–419.
7 Yan Z, Fischer K: Always under construction – Dynamic variations in adult cognitive microdevelopment. Hum Dev 2002;45:141–160.
8 Baltes MM, Kuehl KP, Sowarka D: Testing for limits of cognitive reserve capacity: A promising strategy for early diagnosis of dementia? J Gerontol 1992;47:P165–P167.
9 Lindenberger U, Baltes PB: Testing-the-limits and experimental simulation: Two methods to explicate the role of learning in development. Hum Dev 1995;38:349–360.
10 Salthouse TA: The processing-speed theory of adult age differences in cognition. Psychol Rev 1996;103:403–428.
11 Bryk AS, Raudenbush SW: Hierarchical linear models. Newbury Park, Sage, 1992.
12 Goldstein H: Multilevel statistical models, ed 2. London, Arnold, 1995.
13 Baltes MM, Raykov T: Prospective validity of cognitive plasticity in the diagnosis of mental status: A structural equation model. Neuropsychology 1996;10:549–556.
14 Baltes PB, Lindenberger U: On the range of cognitive plasticity in old age as a function of experience: 15 years of intervention research. Behav Ther 1988;19:283–300.
15 Deeg DJH, Knipscheer CPM, Van Tilburg W: Autonomy and well-being in the aging population – Concepts and design of the Longitudinal Aging Study Amsterdam. Bunnik, Nederlands Instituut voor de Gerontologie, 1993.
16 Aartsen MJ, Smits CHM, Van Tilburg T, Knipscheer CPM, Deeg DJH: Activity in older adults: Cause or consequence of cognitive functioning? A longitudinal study on everyday activities and cognitive performance in older adults. J Gerontol B Psychol Sci Soc Sci 2002; 57B:P153–P162.
17 Ogden WC, Martin DW, Paap KR: Processing demands of encoding: What does secondary task performance reflect? J Exp Psychol 1980; 6:355–367.
18 Neale MC, Boker SM, Xie G, Maes HH: Mx Statistical Modeling, ed 6. Richmond, VCU, Department of Psychiatry, 2002.
19 MacCallum R, Browne M, Sugawara HM: Power analysis and determination of sample size for covariance structure modeling. Psychol Methods 1996;2:130–149.
20 Nevitt J, Hancock GR: Performance of bootstrapping approaches to model test statistics and parameter standard error estimation in structural equation modeling. Struct Equation Model 2001;8:353–377.

Gerontology

Gerontology 2004;50:22–27
DOI: 10.1159/000074385

Age Differences in the Heritability of Mean and Intraindividual Variation of Psychological Distress

Michelle Neiss[a] David M. Almeida[b]

[a]University of Southampton, Southampton, UK, and [b]Human Development and Family Studies, Pennsylvania State University, State College, Pa., USA

Key Words

Negative affect · Behavioral genetics · Intraindividual variation · Emotion regulation

Abstract

Background: An important question in the study of intraindividual variability is whether the same explanatory mechanisms govern between person variation and within person variation. ***Objective:*** This paper investigates genetic and environmental influences on affect across varying time frames and genetic and environmental influences on within person variation in affect. ***Methods:*** Twin participants aged 25–74 years provided information on their affective experiences over monthly, weekly, and daily recall periods. Questionnaires and daily telephone interviews were used to assess frequency of negative emotions. ***Results:*** Monthly, weekly, and daily reports of negative affect all showed modest genetic influence. Monthly and daily measures also demonstrated modest shared environmental influence. Sibling resemblance in within-person variation in affect was accounted for entirely by shared environment. Tests for age differences in magnitude of genetic and environmental effects revealed that genetic influences on monthly reports of affect were greater among older adults, but genetic influences on daily affective experiences were lower among older adults. ***Conclusions:*** Lowered heritability in daily affect among older adults contradicts standard behavior genetic expectations, and is consistent with the proposition that older adults gain skills in emotion regulation.

An important question in the study of intraindividual variability is whether the same explanatory mechanisms govern between person variation and within person variation. When this is the case the phenomenon is considered to have a property of ergodicity. For certain phenomena this property is unlikely [1]. For example, between-person differences reflected by mean levels of emotions may represent emotional set points and are likely to be influenced by genetically based dispositions whereas fluctuations around such set points (i.e. intraindividual variations) are more influenced by environmental conditions [2].

This paper uses a behavior genetic design to inform us about dispositional and environmental influences on negative affect within a life span framework. While substantial evidence suggests that negative mood is influenced by genetic factors [3, 4], few studies have investigated age differences in heritability. We investigate environmental and genetic influences on monthly, weekly, and daily

KARGER

Fax + 41 61 306 12 34
E-Mail karger@karger.ch
www.karger.com

0304–324X/04/0501–0022$21.00/0

Accessible online at:
www.karger.com/ger

Prof. Dave Almeida
Pennsylvania State University, Gerontology Center
135 E. Nittany Avenue, Suite 405
State College, PA 16801-5363 (USA)
Tel. +1 814 865 3252, Fax +1 814 863 9423, E-Mail almeida@psu.edu

reports of negative affect. A focus on differing time frames allows us to compare more molar time referents (i.e. monthly) that may reflect personality factors with more micro time referents (i.e., daily and weekly) that may reflect more situational and contextual influences on affect. The study also looks at intraindividual variability of daily affect. Using daily reports of negative mood, our diary design allows us to examine environmental and genetic sources of fluctuation in mood.

Our study was sparked by interest in the idea that people gain skills in emotional regulation as they age. Research suggests that older people report lower levels of negative affect [5]; a finding that is sometimes interpreted as indirect evidence of developmental gains in the ability to regulate emotions [5, 6]. An alternative explanation, however, is that affect primarily reflects innate disposition and what is often interpreted as emotional regulation is in fact a genotype → environment effect [7]. Scarr's [7] work on intelligence, for example, shows increasing heritability for intelligence over time, which she interprets as evidence that people are selecting opportunities or contexts based on their interests and talents.

Gene → environment effects highlight potential correlations between persons and their environments, such that people with more negative emotional dispositions experience more negative environments. This may reflect active gene-environment correlation, whereby people with greater temperamental positive affectivity are more likely to choose social partners or contexts that maintain relatively positive emotions. Gene–environment correlation can also reflect more evocative effects. Some temperamental styles may facilitate the development of positive relationships, whereas other styles may inhibit the development of relationships. For example, some people with depressive symptoms engage in excessive reassurance seeking, which leads to greater interpersonal rejection, which in turn can lead to greater depression [8]. Over time, therefore, we might see that environments covary with and amplify the effect of initial genetic differences between people. If so, the cumulative effect of genetic differences on emotional experiences may lead to higher heritability estimates among older adults.

In contrast to the dispositional viewpoint, theories concerning age and emotional regulation suggest that older adults are better able generally to control their emotions. This explanation relies less on individual differences, which are potentially under genetic influence, than on general developmental gains. Labouvie-Vief and her colleagues have suggested that in adulthood, people reintegrate affective awareness into their cognitive understanding [9]. In support of her theory, adults were found to have significantly higher levels of emotional understanding and control when compared to adolescents. Other researchers have also found evidence of increased emotional regulation among older adults [5, 10]. Gross et al. [10] found that older adults across diverse cultural and social groups reported greater emotional control than younger adults, suggesting that this gain is a general developmental change. If people acquire generally the ability to control more effectively their emotions, this developmental gain is independent of personality. To the extent that personality is heritable, we would thus expect genetic effects to decrease over time. The purpose of this study is to examine age differences in heritability estimates as a way of investigating whether affect among older adults seems to be more reflective of innate temperament or whether there is evidence of developmental changes in the source of between-person and within-person variation.

Method

Sample and Procedure

Data for the analyses are from the National Study of Daily Experiences (NSDE), one of the in-depth studies that are part of the National Survey of Midlife in the United States Survey (MIDUS) carried out under the auspices of the John D. and Catherine T. MacArthur Foundation Research Network on Successful Midlife. The total NSDE sample of 1,483 is comprised of 1,031 randomly selected respondents from the MIDUS random digit dialed (RDD) subsample and 452 MIDUS twins. We selected twins if twin pairs had high self-reported certainty of zygosity. For the present analysis we used 210 same-sex twin pairs: 111 identical or monozygotic (MZ) pairs, 99 fraternal or dizygotic (DZ) pairs.

Twins ranged in age from 25 to 74 years. Forty-seven percent of the respondents were male, 53% were female. The majority (76%) of respondents were married, 9% were divorced, 2% were separated, 2% were widowed, and 11% were never-married. Respondents were primarily white (92%). Six percent of the respondents were African American. Seventy-seven percent of the respondents were currently working, while 6% were retired.

Over the course of eight consecutive evenings, respondents completed short telephone interviews about their daily experiences. On the final evening of interviewing, respondents also answered several questions about their previous week. To aid independence of reporting, co-twins were interviewed at least two weeks apart. The initiation of interviews was staggered across the day of the week to control for the possible confounding between day of study and day of week.

Negative Affect

Our analyses make use of four measures of negative affect that differ in interval of recall and in level of aggregation. Each affect measure used an inventory of emotions from the Non-Specific Psychological Distress Scale [11]. The scale includes emotions such as sadness, hopelessness, anxiety, and restlessness. Respondents indicated how much of the time they experienced each emotion on a

Table 1. Age differences and sibling resemblance for negative affect variables

Negative affect variable	Younger		Older		t	MZ pairs, r	DZ pairs, r
	mean	SD	mean	SD			
Monthly recall	0.16	0.15	0.14	0.13	–1.99*	0.18	0.14
Weekly recall	0.10	0.10	0.07	0.09	–3.20**	0.22*	0.04
Daily recall	0.06	0.07	0.04	0.05	–4.00***	0.29**	0.13
Intraindividual variation	0.07	0.06	0.05	0.05	–3.90***	0.21*	0.27**

* $p < 0.05$; ** $p < 0.01$; *** $p < 0.001$.

5-point scale from *none of the time* to *all of the time*. For each of the following measures of negative affect, mean scores across these items were calculated.

Monthly negative affect: during the initial baseline MIDUS data collection, respondents indicated how often they felt each of 6 emotions 'during the past thirty days' (Cronbach's alpha = 0.87). *Weekly negative affect* was assessed at the conclusion of the final day of interviewing, when respondents were asked how often they felt each of 10 emotions 'during the past week' (Cronbach's alpha = 0.85). *Daily negative affect:* during the daily telephone interviews, respondents indicated how often they felt each of 10 emotions 'during the past 24 hours'. A daily aggregate measure was created by computing the mean of the daily reports across the eight diary days (Cronbach's alpha = 0.90). *Intraindividual variation in negative affect* was measured by calculating the within person standard deviation of the daily negative affect scores across the 8 diary days. This score represents an individual's fluctuation of daily negative affect.

Results

Preliminary Analyses

Inspection of our variables revealed the presence of extreme values (z-scores >4). We used a log transformation to reduce the influence of outliers for all four variables. The daily affect scores for two individuals remained quite extreme (z-scores >5) after these transformations. We recoded these extreme values to missing.

Age and gender effects can serve to increase twin resemblance, which may be problematic when estimating genetic and environmental influences. Age was related significantly to all affect variables ($r_{monthly} = -0.17$, $p < 0.001$; $r_{weekly} = -0.14$, $p < 0.01$; $r_{daily} = -0.14$, $p < 0.01$), such that older adults tended to have lower levels of negative affect regardless of time frame. Older adults also reported less variability in daily affective ratings as compared to younger adults ($r = -0.15$, $p < 0.01$). Table 1 displays the age differences by providing the means and standard deviations for each of the affect variables for younger and older participants. The younger group (101 pairs) consisted of people whose ages ranged from 25 to 40. The older group (109 pairs) contained people age 41 and over. Respondents, on average, reported greater levels of negative affect when asked to recall over the entire week as compared to the aggregate of daily reports of negative affect across that same week. The discrepancy between the daily measure and the weekly measure suggested that respondents tended to overestimate the frequency of negative affect when they recalled their emotions over longer time intervals.

Significant gender effects were also present. Women reported higher levels of negative affect at the weekly ($t = -2.11$, $p < 0.05$) and daily ($t = -2.39$, $p < 0.05$) levels. Women also reported greater variability in daily affective ratings ($t = -3.98$, $p < 0.001$). Given these main effects, we controlled all four affect variables for both age and gender at the individual level. We then standardized each variable.

Sibling Correlations

In the first step of the behavior genetic analysis we computed the within-sibling correlations for each of the four variables (table 1). For the first three measures, the correlations for the identical twins were slightly to moderately higher than the correlations for the fraternal twins, indicating some genetic influence for the mean level of negative affect. For intraindividual variability in affect, however, the correlation among fraternal twins was actually higher than that among identical twins. This pattern suggests twin resemblance for variability in affect can be attributed to shared environment and that genetic factors do not explain individual differences in intraindividual variability.

Structural Equation Modeling

To obtain estimates of genetic and environmental influences on negative affect, we conducted a series of

Table 2. Model fitting results

Negative affect variable	χ^2	p	d.f.	RMSEA	AIC	Proportion of variance		
						a^2	c^2	e^2
Monthly	0.68	0.88	3	0.000	–5.32	0.09	0.10	0.82
Weekly	1.11	0.77	3	0.000	–4.89	0.20	0.00	0.80
Daily	2.60	0.46	3	0.018	–3.40	0.14	0.15	0.71
Intraindividual variation	4.52	0.21	3	0.053	–1.48	0.00	0.24	0.76

Table 3. Model fitting results for age-difference model in daily negative affect

Negative affect	χ^2	d.f.	p	RMSEA	AIC	a^2	c^2	e^2
Monthly	7.84	6	0.25	0.085	–4.16			
Younger people						0.00	0.24	0.76
Older people						0.13	0.00	0.87
Daily	6.68	6	0.35	0.037	–5.32			
Younger people						0.20	0.23	0.57
Older people						0.00	0.09	0.91

Structural Equations Models via the Mx program [12]. This procedure allowed us to decompose the observed variance in each of the variables into three factors: Additive genetic influences (a), shared environmental influences (c), and non-shared environmental influences (e). Genetic influences accounted for between 9 and 20% of the variance in mean levels of negative affect. Shared environmental influences accounted for minimal variance in the mean levels weekly negative affect, but had a modest effect on both monthly and daily affect. The largest share of variance in all models was attributable to unique (non-shared) environmental influences. The last row in table 2 shows the results for intraindividual variation. Shared environmental influences accounted for 24% of the variance in daily mood, whereas genetic influences were minimal. Again, non-shared environment accounted for a substantial portion of the variance (74%).

Age Differences

The final set of analyses assessed age differences in the magnitudes of genetic and environmental influences in the previous models. We compared models that constrained parameters to be equal across the age groups with models that allowed parameters for younger twin pairs to differ from older pairs. This allowed us to see whether observed phenotypic variance within each group can be differentially apportioned.

A model in which parameters differed across the two age groups fit better than one in which genetic and environmental estimates were constrained to be equal for both monthly and daily levels of negative affect. Model fitting results and parameter estimates for the age difference models are provided in table 3. For monthly levels of negative affect, the pattern follows the standard behavioral genetic prediction: genetic influences are larger among older adults as compared to younger adults. In addition, shared environmental influences are stronger among younger adults. A different pattern emerges for daily levels of negative affect; however, heritability is larger among younger adults than among older adults, as is shared environment.

Discussion

The results of these analyses suggest three findings. First, regardless of time frame, mean level of negative affect is partially heritable. This finding is consistent with prior studies noting significant heritability for depression [13] and negative affect [3]. Our results provide evidence that genetic influences can account for individual differences in general affective tendencies and in day-to-day negative mood. Second, evidence for shared environment was found for monthly and daily levels of negative mood, as well as variation in daily mood. Shared environment among these adult twins may be reflective of daily events or stressors that revolve around the family. In addition, the role of shared environment in negative affect may reflect parental socialization concerning emotion. Eisenberg, Cumberland, and Spinrad [14] note that emotional socialization may focus particularly on negative emotions. Third, for both age groups, there was no evidence for genetic influences on intraindividual variation. Shared environmental influences, however, were sizeable. This finding supports the set point theory [2]: baseline or average mood is heritable, while fluctuations around that set point are primarily due to environmental events.

Age differences in genetic and environmental effects were present for monthly and daily affect. Genetic influences explained more of the variance in older adults' monthly affect, and shared environmental influences explained less, as compared to younger adults. This pattern followed the dispositional viewpoint, with genetic effects amplified over time. Daily affect, however, revealed a different pattern of results. Shared environmental estimates were again higher among younger adults. This finding is not surprising, reflecting greater temporal proximity to the shared rearing environment. The absence of genetic influence on affect among older adults, however, fails to confirm the dispositional viewpoint. Overall, the pattern supports the idea that temperament is no longer as strong a predictor of differences in day-to-day negative affect among older adults. While the cross-sectional nature of the study does not allow us to interpret this as an age change, the finding is consistent with the concept of developmental gains in emotional regulation.

How can we reconcile the disparate patterns for daily and monthly affect? We suggest that this difference arises, in part, because monthly and daily measures of affect assess different aspects of affective experience. Prior research has shown that people tend to overestimate the intensity of emotions over longer time frames [15, 16] and tend to rely on most recent (end) and peak affective experiences when recalling retrospectively [17, 18]. Our respondents demonstrated a similar pattern, recalling greater frequency of negative affect over the past week than indicated by their actual daily experiences. Perhaps some of the genetic effect on affect is unique to the experience of particularly intense or frequent negative emotions, which serve to bias people's recall.

It should be noted that while we can test whether sources of variance differ between age groups, we cannot explain mean-level differences between groups using our basic behavior genetic model. Nevertheless, significant age differences in the proportion of variance attributed to genetic and environmental influences provide a unique perspective on developmental changes. Our findings highlight two divergent patterns, with differing implications. In the case of monthly affect, heritability was greater among older adults. The next step is to understand how this difference develops. Is it an age-related change? What environments or experiences can account for an amplification of genetic effects over time? In the case of daily affect, heritability was lower among older adults. Decreased heritability over time calls for its own unique developmental explanation. We suggest that this pattern is consistent with the idea that people gain emotional regulation skills over time, but this connection should be explored explicitly in future research. Younger adults had higher levels of daily affect, and a greater portion of the differences among younger adults in daily affect was attributable to genetic effects. Overall, our findings suggest that temperament plays less of a role in explaining between-person differences in day-to-day affect as we age. A decline in the role of temperament can be explained by a general developmental gain in emotional regulation that is independent of personality or innate factors.

Acknowledgment

This project was supported by the John D. and Catherine T. MacArthur Foundation Research Network on Successful Midlife Development, the W.K. Kellogg Foundation, the Alfred P. Sloan Foundation and grants from the National Institute of Mental Health (MH53372) and the National Institute on Aging (AG16731).

References

1 Molenaar PCM, Huizenga HM, Nesselroade JR: The relationship between the structure of inter-individual and intra-individual variability: A theoretical and empirical vindication of developmental system theory; in Staudinger UM, Lindenberger U (eds): Understanding Human Development: Dialogues with Lifespan Psychology. Dordrecht, Kluwer, 2003, pp 339–360.
2 Lykken D, Tellegen A: Happiness is a stochastic phenomenon. Psychol Sci 1996;7:186–189.
3 Baker LA, Cesa IL, Gatz, M, Mellins C: Genetic and environmental influences on positive and negative affect: Support for a two-factor theory. Psych Aging 1992;7:158–163.
4 Gatz M, Pedersen NL, Plomin R, Nesselroade JR, McClearn GE: Importance of shared genes and shared environments for symptoms of depression in older adults. J Abnormal Psych 1992;101:701–708.
5 Lawton MP, Kleban MH, Rajagopal D, Dean J: Dimensions of affective experience in three age groups. Psych Aging 1992;7:171–184.
6 Carstensen LL, Isaacowitz DM, Charles ST: Taking time seriously: A theory of socioemotional selectivity. Am Psychol 1999;54:165–181.
7 Scarr S: Biological and cultural diversity: The legacy of Darwin for development. Child Dev 1993;64:1333–1353.
8 Joiner TE, Metalsky GI, Katz J, Beach SRH: Depression and excessive reassurance-seeking. Psychol Inquiry 1999;10:269–278.
9 Labouvie-Vief G, Hakim-Larson J, DeVoe M, Schoeberlein S: Emotions and self-regulation: A life span view. Human Dev 1989;32:279–299.
10 Gross JJ, Carstensen LL, Pasupathi M, Tsai J, Gotestam Skorpen C, Hsu AYC: Emotion and aging: Experience, expression, and control. Psych Aging 1997;12:590–599.
11 Mroczek DK, Kolarz CM: The effect of age on positive and negative affect: A developmental perspective on happiness. J Pers Social Psych 1998;75:1333–1349.
12 Neale MC: Mx: Statistical Modeling, ed 4. Richmond, Department of Psychiatry, 1997.
13 McGue M, Christensen K: Genetic and environmental contributions to depression symptomatology: Evidence from Danish twins 75 years of age and older. J Abnormal Psych 1997;106:439–448.
14 Eisenberg N, Cumberland A, Spinrad TL: Parental socialization of emotion. Psychol Inquiry 1998;9:241–273.
15 Parkinson B, Briner RB, Reynolds S, Totterdell P: Time frames for mood: Relations between momentary and generalized ratings of affect. Pers Social Psych Bull 1995;21:331–339.
16 Thomas DL, Diener E: Memory accuracy in the recall of emotions. J Pers Social Psych 1990;59:291–297.
17 Kahneman D: Objective happiness; in Kahneman D, Diener E, Schwartz N (eds): Well-Being: The Foundations of Hedonic Psychology. New York, Russell Sage Foundation, 1999, pp 1–25.
18 Redelmeier D, Kahneman D: Patients' memories of painful medical treatments: Real-time and retrospective evaluations of two minimally invasive procedures. Pain 1996;116:3–8.

Gerontology

Gerontology 2004;50:28–34
DOI: 10.1159/000074386

Aging and Attenuated Processing Robustness

Evidence from Cognitive and Sensorimotor Functioning

Shu-Chen Li Oliver Huxhold Florian Schmiedek

Center for Lifespan Psychology, Max Planck Institute for Human Development, Berlin, Germany

Key Words
Cognitive aging · Sensorimotor functioning · Intraindividual variability · Neuronal noise · Processing fidelity

Abstract
Background: Within-person, across-time variations in processes and performance are intrinsic to all aspects of human functioning. ***Objective:*** This article starts with a brief taxonomy of intraindividual dynamics. There are adaptive as well as non-adaptive types of intraindividual variations that unfold with different degrees of reversibility on different time scales and involve either single, or systems of, functions. ***Methods:*** Empirical findings regarding aging and a specific type of intraindividual variation, namely attenuated processing robustness, are then presented with respect to cognitive and sensorimotor functioning. ***Results:*** In both domains of functioning, old adults exhibit less robust functioning with a greater amount of week-to-week, day-to-day, or trial-by-trial fluctuations in their cognitive, walking, and postural control performances. ***Conclusion:*** Currently, the causes for the attenuation of processing robustness in cognitive and sensorimotor functioning are not well understood. Neurocomputational models are useful tools for exploring the tripartite relationships between the aging of neural information-processing fidelity, and cognitive, and sensorimotor processes.

Variability is inherent in the processes of any self-organizing dynamic system. Humans are self-constructing living systems [1]; hence, intraindividual variability is intrinsic to all aspects of human functioning. While issues on between-individual differences in performance levels have been the focus of different research orientations (e.g. experimental and differential approaches), much less is known about intraindividual variations and interindividual differences of intraindividual variations. Previously, the term, 'intraindividual variability', had been defined as short-term, reversible within-individual changes that represents a steady state 'hum' of an individual [2]. To differentiate between this type of variability and many other types of intraindividual variations, here we take 'intraindividual dynamics' as a broad, superordinate concept that can be further classified. We define 'intraindividual dynamics' as: variations and transformations in an individual's processes or performance over time that are

KARGER

Fax + 41 61 306 12 34
E-Mail karger@karger.ch
www.karger.com

0304–324X/04/0501–0028$21.00/0

Accessible online at:
www.karger.com/ger

Shu-Chen Li
Center for Lifespan Psychology, Max Planck Institute for Human Development
Lentzeallee 94
DE–14195 Berlin (Germany)
Tel. +49 30 82406 305, Fax +49 30 82499 39, E-Mail Shuchen@mpib-berlin.mpg.de

produced by endogenous factors (e.g. neurobiological and cognitive processes) and their interactions with contextual and experiential influences.

A Taxonomy of Intraindividual Dynamics

Different types of intraindividual variation unfold with different degrees of reversibility on different time scales and involve either single or multiple functions. As Ford [1] pointed out, although 'being' (functioning) and 'becoming' (developing throughout the lifespan or ontogeny) are related, they are also distinct. It is, therefore, important to differentiate between short-term, relatively reversible variations in functioning and progressive long-term, relatively permanent lifespan developmental changes. Moreover, the concept of intraindividual dynamics should not be limited only to variations within a given specific function; rather, it also applies to transformations in the functional organization of related functions. Considered jointly, these two vantage points (i.e. functioning and developing) give rise to four broad categories of intraindividudal dynamics (see summary in fig. 1a).

Relatively permanent *intraindividual changes* in physical growth, cognitive development, and cognitive aging are all examples of the developing type of intraindividual dynamics that cumulatively unfold on relatively long-term time scales (e.g. across months, years, and decades). Besides the univariate phenomena of intraindividual changes within each of the specific functions, developmental or aging-related transformations in the functional organization of mental abilities, cognitive processes, as well as sensorimotor processes are expressed on the multivariate level. With only a few exceptions on aging and the dedifferentiation of ability structure [3–5], longitudinal data addressing transformations in the functional organizations of processes or abilities either at the neuronal or behavioral level are rare. However, available cross-sectional approximations – specifically, empirical evidence of developmental neuronal specification [6], aging-related alterations in neural circuitry [7, 8] and the differentiation-dedifferentiation of ability structure across the lifespan [9, 10] – all indicate that future longitudinal research on intraindividual dynamics regarding the organization of system of functions are necessary.

Aside from intraindividual changes occurring across months, years, or decades, there are other types of relatively more reversible intraindividual variations that unfold on time scales of testing trials, training sessions, or weeks. Ford [1] termed these as the 'being' type of intraindividual variability, and primarily emphasized cyclic variations within limits that could be characterized as the steady metabolic rhythms of the individual (e.g., neuronal firing rate, hormonal secretions, or heart rate). Besides such cyclic, rhythmic variations, there could also be what we term the 'functioning' type of short-term intraindividual variations that are related to the processing aspect of behavior and performance, such as random processing fluctuation – or lack of processing robustness – around asymptotic functioning [10, 11], as well as functional plasticity, diversity, and adaptability. Functional plasticity refers to the amount of training gain an individual derives from relatively short-term but intensive training on a given task. Most cognitive training research found that, even in old age, individuals are still able to benefit from intensive practice and training [12, 13]. Functional diversity signifies digressions of functioning that may be associated with exploratory behavior and strategies during the initial acquisition of complex new tasks [cf. 14, 15]. For instance, recently it was found that before performance asymptotes were reached, intraindividual variations during the acquisition phase of learning an array of cognitive tasks (e.g. reasoning, perceptual speed, and memory) correlated positively with performance level [16]. In a complex spatial memory task where individuals might engage in exploring different strategies when performing the task, intraindividual week-to-week variations were also found to correlate positively with performance level [11]. Functional adaptability indicates an individual's ability to alter functioning when faced with perturbations in the human-task environment – either due, indeed, to sudden fluctuations in processing (e.g., an attention blink) or more demanding task requirements – in order to regain maximum functioning.

The above classification of intraindividual dynamics allows the distinctions between adaptive and non-adaptive types of intraindividual variations to be more readily made on a priori theoretical grounds (see fig. 1b for a schematization of the distinctions). For any given self-organizing organism or system, random processing fluctuation around a given maximum level of functioning after the asymptote is reached indicates a lack of processing robustness and can be expected to be non-adaptive. In contrast, the functional plasticity of organisms (or systems) to obtain large learning gains after some exposure to a task, the diversity of their exploratory behavior and strategies when acquiring a complex task, or their adaptability to quickly recover a high level of functioning when conditions for maximum functioning are challenged can

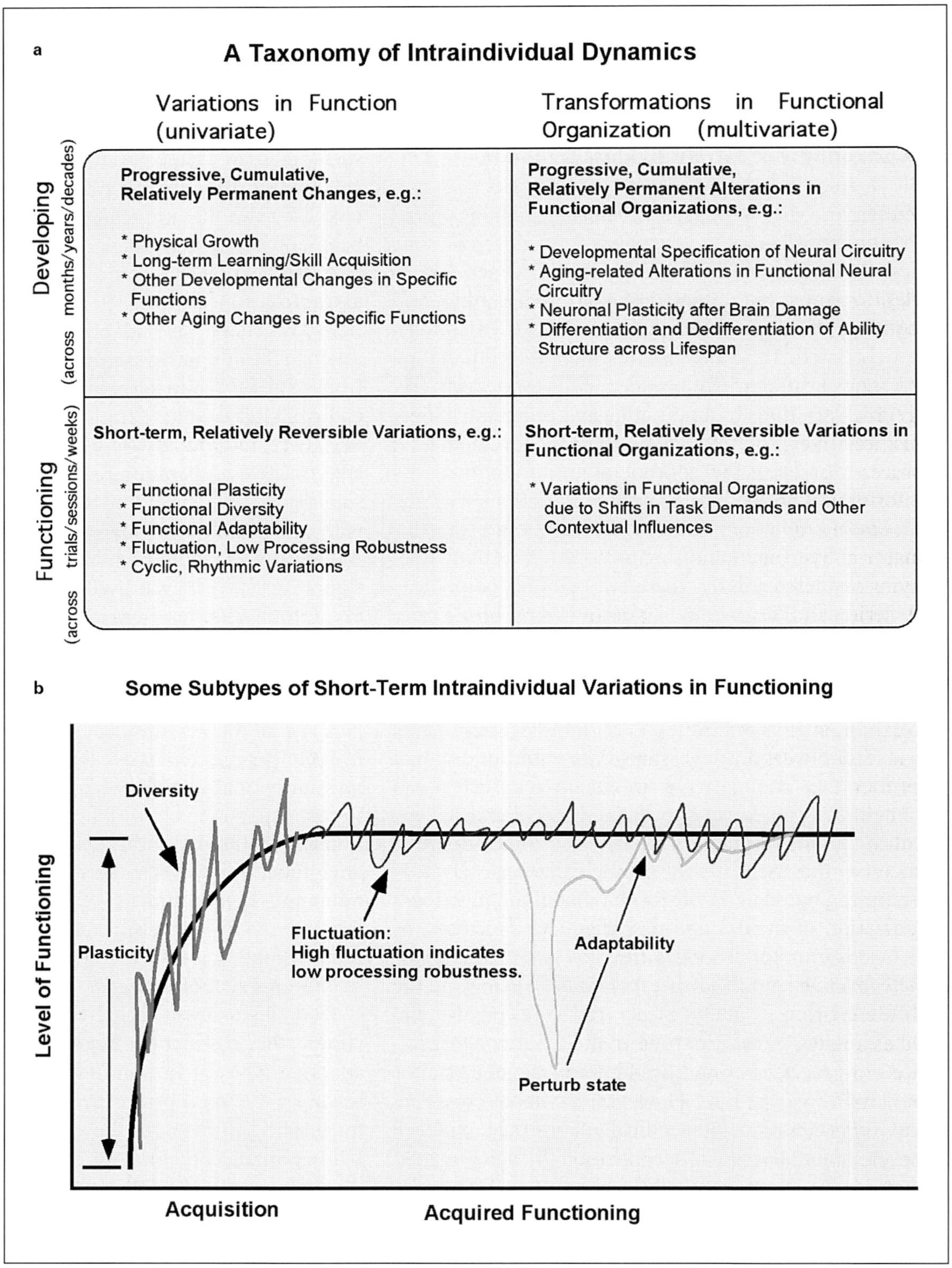

Fig. 1. Classifications of intraindividual dynamics. **a** A taxonomy of intraindividual dynamics. **b** Differentiating between subtypes of short-term intraindividual variations in functioning.

all be expected to be adaptive. Lastly, there are currently no clear, direct empirical data on short-term transformations in the functional organization of abilities and processes that are due to, for instance, the individual's response to shifts in environmental or task conditions. However, this type of intraindividual variation is conceptually distinct from other aspects of intraindividual dynamics, and merits future empirical investigations.

Aging and Attenuated Processing Robustness of Cognitive Functioning

This article focuses only on one specific aspect of intraindividual dynamics, namely the extent of processing robustness. Besides speed and accuracy per se, the extent of processing robustness reflects another important aspect of information processing. In many cognitive tasks, a lack of processing robustness could be indicated by intraindividual trial-by-trial reaction time (RT) fluctuations when carrying out a given task across multiple trials.

A series of recent studies examined intraindividual trial-by-trial RT fluctuations in old people. Rabbitt et al. [17] measured both trial-by-trial and week-to-week fluctuations in old people's RTs across 36 weeks. Individuals who exhibited greater within-session trial-by-trial and between-session week-to-week variability when performing letter identification tasks also scored lower on a culture-fair intelligence test. Another study explored the diagnostic utility of trial-by-trial RT variability in predicting aging-related pathology, and found that independent of mean performance, trial-by-trial RT fluctuations uniquely contributed to predicting dementia group membership [18]. We examined intraindividual RT fluctuations in a lifespan sample covering the age range from 6 to 89 years [10]. Here processing robustness was operationally defined as a reflected measure based on the summary composite score of intraindividual RT fluctuations of a battery of cognitive tasks. The tasks measured the reaction times of processes, such as visual search, response competition, memory search, and choice decision. Results from variance component analyses showed that, in late adulthood and old age, processing robustness added at least as much unique variance as processing speed in predicting fluid intelligence. Moreover, processing robustness predicted old people's chronological age above and beyond processing speed. Interestingly, all these effects were unique to the senescence portion of the lifespan.

Aging and Attenuated Processing Robustness of Sensorimotor Functioning

Besides the interest in the processing robustness of cognitive functioning, robustness in old people's sensorimotor functioning has also attracted research attention. In one study, short-term fluctuations in elderly people's sensorimotor performance were investigated by biweekly measures of walking and turning tasks across 7 months [11]. Across the age range from 64 to 86 years, it was found that increased biweekly intraindividual fluctuation in sensorimotor performance, indicating less robust sensorimotor functioning, was related to increasing age (average correlation 0.44) and a lower level of sensorimotor functioning (average correlation –0.78 after the effect of age was partialed out). Moreover, there was a cross-domain association: independent of their mean performances, the individuals who lacked processing robustness in sensorimotor functioning also showed worse text and spatial memory. For instance, within-individual week-to-week fluctuations in walking steps added 18 and 9% unique variance in predicting text and spatial memory, respectively.

Lacking Processing Robustness in Terms of Increased Moment-to-Moment Postural Sway

Moment-to-moment postural sway has also been used to examine aging and the attenuation of processing robustness in sensorimotor functioning. Old people tend to sway more than young adults under various conditions [19]. Postural sway is commonly measured by the force platform and is indexed by the drift of the center of pressure (COP), which results from all forces the individual applies on the platform in order to maintain the upright posture. The total COP drift traveled within a given trial duration (COP area) is a summary measure of the amount of sway exhibited in a given trial. The COP area thus could serve as an overall index for the degree of processing robustness of the postural control system [see also 20].

Rarely has the question regarding trial-by-trial or session-by-session fluctuations in postural sway been asked. Example data illustrating these two aspects of processing robustness in sensorimotor functioning were taken from one young and one old adult. Their dynamic posturography was measured by a computerized force platform under various conditions across 12 successive sessions with a 3-day inter-session interval. After a practice session, sessions 2–10 and 11–12 were devoted to the examinations of day-to-day and trial-by-trial fluctuations in postural sway under various conditions. Specifically, the

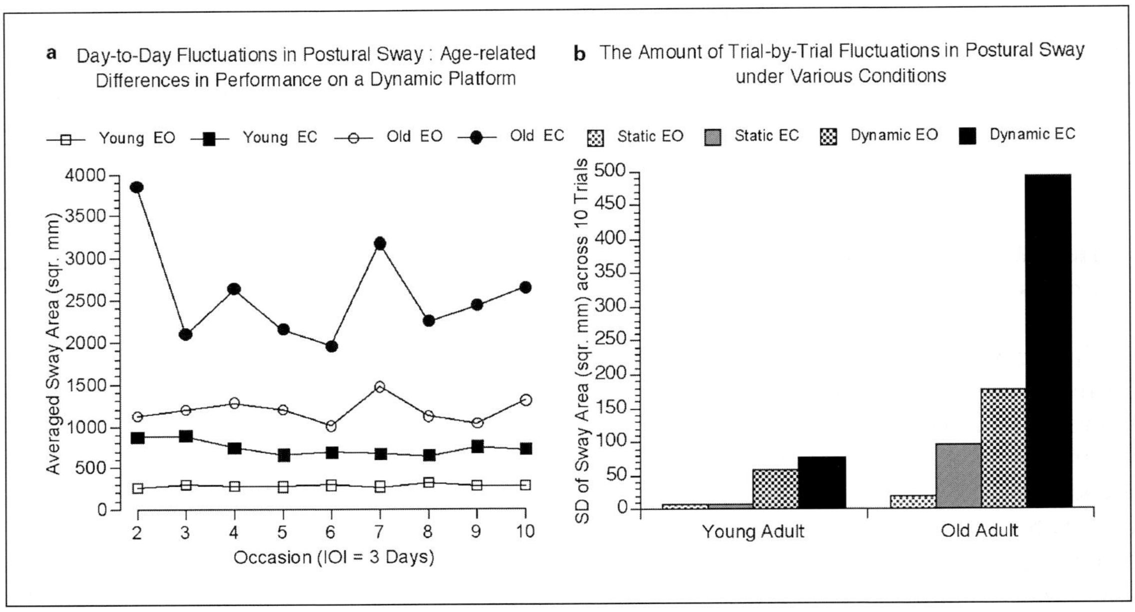

Fig. 2. Processing robustness of sensorimotor functioning measured in terms of postural sway. **a** Day-to-day fluctuations in sensorimotor functioning of an old adult and a young adult are compared with respect to postural sway measured on a dynamic platform under eyes-open (EO) and eyes-closed (EC) conditions. **b** The amount of the trial-by-trial fluctuations in postural sway of an old adult and a young adult across ten successive trials (expressed as the standard deviation of sway area) were compared in four experimental conditions: static platform eyes-open (Static EO), static platform eyes-closed (Static EC), dynamic platform EO (dynamic EO), and dynamic platform EC (dynamic EC).

experimental demands were designed to challenge the efficacy of the dynamic postural control system (with the platform moving three degrees up and down in a sinusoidal fashion) by removing visual input in the eyes-closed (EC) condition as opposed to the eyes-open (EO) control condition (sessions 2–10). Sessions 11 and 12 further compared the system to adapt to a dynamic (i.e. moving) platform or the static control condition, under EO and EC conditions. Body sway in each of these conditions was measured four times in a given session to improve measurement reliability.

Regarding day-to-day fluctuations, figure 2a shows the patterns of variation in the averaged COP area for sessions 2–10. The results clearly showed that whereas the young adult exhibited a relatively stable performance across sessions, the average sway of the old adult varied much more from day to day. More interestingly, this age-related difference in day-to-day fluctuations was more pronounced under the more demanding EC condition, which challenged the postural system by removing visual input.

Regarding trial-by-trial fluctuations, figure 2b exemplifies the standard deviation of the sway areas across ten trials in a given session. It is readily seen that, overall, the amount of trial-by-trial fluctuations in sway is a function of how much the postural system is challenged by perturbing the sensory inputs. For both young and old adults, the SD of trial-by-trial sway was larger in the more demanding dynamic conditions. Furthermore, the data suggested that the old adult's postural system was more affected than that of the young adult by the various sensory constraints. For example, removing visual input under the easier, static condition did not disturb the young postural system at all, but the old adult clearly swayed much more with closed eyes. The results also highlight the effect of visual input on old adult's postural control. The increased trial-by-trial fluctuations in sway produced by simply asking the old adult to close the eyes while standing on the *static* platform (an increase of 75.5 mm^2 in the SD of sway area) is much greater than that produced by the more demanding, dynamic condition observed in the young (an effect of 20 mm^2). Moreover, for the old adult the further need to adapt to a dynamic platform increased the trial-by-trial fluctuations in sway even more. In the most demanding condition with eyes closed while standing on the dynamic platform, the amount of trial-by-trial fluctuations in sway was about five times higher than that of the young adult.

Neural Correlates of Attenuated Processing Robustness: A Neurocomputational View

The empirical findings reviewed thus far suggest that decreased processing robustness in old age is of theoretical relevance to the neuronal noise hypothesis of aging [21]. A recent neurocomputational theory provides a cross-level account that links aging-related deficits in neuromodulation with increased neuronal noise, which, in turn, has subsequent effects on representational distinctiveness, and a variety of cognitive aging phenomena, including increased intraindividual performance fluctuation and ability dedifferentiation [22]. Details of how reduced signal transmission fidelity at the neuronal level might decrease processing robustness observed at the information-processing and behavioral levels are mostly unknown. However, neurocomputational simulations suggest some possible theoretical considerations, beyond the scope of this paper.

Conclusion and Outlook

Attenuated processing robustness is a subtype of intraindividual dynamics that is mostly non-adaptive. Current evidence indicates that this type of intraindividual variation in cognitive functioning is positively related with advancing old age, negatively related to intellectual performance, and predictive of old-age related brain pathology. Neurocomputational simulations suggest that aging-related decline in neuromodulation could be a contributing source for attenuated processing robustness in old age. Furthermore, there is also evidence for aging-related decline in the sensorimotor processing robustness, either with respect to walking or postural control. Challenging the postural control system by perturbing the visual or (and) somatosensory inputs increased the amount of trial-by-trial fluctuations in sway of an old adult much more than of a young adult.

Although, thus far most neurcomputational models of aging have focused either on cognitive or sensorimotor phenomena separately, sensorimotor and cognitive processes may not be as segregated as previously thought. Theories of motor learning and postural control postulate that these processes involve complex and dynamic neural computation integrating multiple sensory inputs and motor commands, and that attentional and executive cognitive control processes may be implicated in the integration process. Given the seeming involvement of neuromodulation in aging of both cognitive and sensorimotor systems, large-scale networks with sub-modules capturing cortical functional circuitry for both could serve as general neurocomputational frameworks for exploring the interactions further [22, 23] as contributors to both individual differences in performance level or intraindividual variation.

References

1 Ford DH: Humans as Self-Constructing Living Systems: A Developmental Perspective on Behavior and Personality. Hillsdale, Erlbaum, 1987.

2 Nesselroade JR: The warp and the woof of the developmental fabric; in Downs RM, Liben LS, Palermo DS (eds): Visions of Aesthetics, the Environment and Development: The Legacy of Joachim F. Wohlwill. Hillsdale, Erlbaum, 1991, pp 213–240.

3 Schaie KW, Maitland SB, Willis SL, Intrieri RC: Longitudinal invariance of adult psychometric ability factor structures across 7 years. Psychol Aging 1998;12:8–20.

4 Ghisletta P, Lindenberger U: Age-based structural dynamics between perceptual speed and knowledge in the Berlin Aging Study: Direct evidence for ability dedifferentiation with age. Psychol Aging, in press.

5 Anstey KJ, Hofer SM, Luszcz MA: Cross-sectional and longitudinal patterns of dedifferentiation in late-life cognitive and sensory function: The effects of age, ability, attrition, and occasion of measurement. J Exp Psychol Gen 2003;132:470–487.

6 Johnson MH: Functional brain development in humans. Nat Rev Neurosci 2001;2:475–483.

7 Cabeza R: Hemispheric asymmetry reduction in older adults. Psychol Aging 2002;17:85–100.

8 Reuter-Lorenz PA: New visions of the aging mind and brain. Trends Cogn Sci 2002;6:394–400.

9 Baltes PB, Cornelius SW, Spiro A, Nesselroade JR, Willis SL: Integration versus differentiation of fluid/crystallized intelligence in old age. Dev Psychol 1980;6:625–635.

10 Li SC, Lindenberger U, Hommel B, Aschersleben G, Prinz W, Baltes PB: Lifespan transformations in the couplings among intellectual abilities and constituent cognitive processes. Psychol Sci, in press.

11 Li SC, Aggen SH, Nesselroade JR, Baltes PB: Short-term fluctuations in elderly people's sensorimotor functioning predicting text and spatial memory performance: The MacArthur Successful Aging Study. Gerontology 2001;47:100–116.

12 Baltes PB, Kliegl R: Further testing of limits of cognitive plasticity: Negative age differences in a mnemonic skill are robust. Dev Psychol 1992;28:121–125.
13 Singer T, Lindenberger U, Baltes PB: Plasticity of memory for new learning in very old age: A story of major loss? Psychol Aging 2003;18: 306–317.
14 Siegler RS: Cognitive variability: A key to understanding cognitive development. Curr Dir Psychol Sci 1994;3:1–5.
15 Staddon JER: Adaptive Behavior and Learning. New York, Cambridge University Press, 1983.
16 Allaire JC, Marsiske M: Intraindividual variability in cognitive functioning: Is consistency an index of vulnerability? Paper presented at the Cognitive Aging Conference, Atlanta, Ga., April 2002.
17 Rabbitt P, Osman, P, Moore, B, Stollery B: There are stable individual differences in performance variability, both from moment to moment and from day to day. Q J Exp Psychol 2001;54:981–1003.
18 Hultsch DF, MacDonald SWS, Hunter MA, Levy-Bencheton J, Strauss E: Intraindividual variability in cognitive performance in the older adults: Comparison of adults with mild dementia, adults with arthritis, and healthy adults. Neuropsychology 2001;14:588–598.
19 Woollacott MH: Systems contributing to balance disorders in older adults. J Gerontol [A] 2000;55:M424–M428.
20 Krampe RT, Rapp MA, Bondar A, Baltes PB: Selektion, Optimierung und Kompensation in Doppelaufgaben [Selection, optimization, and compensation in dual task]. Nervenarzt, in press.
21 Welford AT: Signal, noise, performance, and age. Hum Factor 1981;23:97–109.
22 Li SC, Lindenberger U, Sikström S: Aging cognition: From neuromodulation to representation. Trends Cogn Sci 2001;5:479–486.
23 Li SC, Sikström S: Integrative neurocomputational perspectives on cognitive aging, neuromodulation, and representation. Neurosci Biobehav [R] 2003;26:795–808.

Gerontology

Gerontology 2004;50:35–38
DOI: 10.1159/000074387

Gender Differences in Level and Change in Cognitive Functioning

Results from the Longitudinal Aging Study Amsterdam

Marja J. Aartsen[a] Mike Martin[b] Daniel Zimprich[b]

[a]Department of Sociology and Social Gerontology, Vrije Universiteit Amsterdam, Amsterdam, The Netherlands;
[b]Department of Gerontopsychology, Institute of Psychology, University of Zurich, Zurich, Switzerland

Key Words
Gender · Age · Cognitive abilities · Latent change models

Abstract
Background: Gender differences in level of cognitive functioning are frequently observed, but little is known about gender differences in rate of decline of cognitive functioning. ***Objective:*** The present study aims to describe variability between and within men and women specified for four different cognitive abilities at baseline, and variability in change in these abilities among men and women over 6 years. ***Methods:*** We started with a study sample of 1,132 men and 1,175 women, with a measurement interval of 3 years. At wave 3 of the study, 1,552 of the respondents from wave 1 were still present. Differences in level and rate of change were estimated with latent change models. ***Results:*** Women have higher levels of memory functioning then men, but no gender differences were observed for speed or non-verbal reasoning changes. ***Conclusion:*** In spite of evidence for a stronger age-related atrophy of the brain structure of men, no gender differences in decline of cognitive functions could be observed.

Introduction

A classical question in research on cognitive ageing is how cognitive functions change within an individual over age and time, and whether these patterns are different from one variable to another [1]. The theory of fluid and crystallized intelligence [2] proposes that cognitive abilities such as non-verbal reasoning, memory, and processing speed – also referred to as fluid intelligence – decline with ageing, whereas acculturated knowledge – also referred to as crystallized intelligence – increases with ageing. Studies evaluating these predictions observe major inter- and intraindividual differences in cognitive functioning [1, 3].

One of the variables possibly accounting for inter- and intraindividual differences in fluid intelligence is gender. Evidence for gender differences in level of functioning comes from a study on the structure of the brain, in which a more pronounced atrophy with advancing age in males than in females [4] was observed, suggesting that women are less vulnerable to age-related changes in cognitive abilities than men. Also studies on the function of the brain observed gender-related differences in level of cognitive functioning. In those studies, women outperform men with respect to memory functioning [5] and speed [6] and men show better results on spatial abilities [6] and reasoning [7]. Based on significant interactions between

KARGER
Fax + 41 61 306 12 34
E-Mail karger@karger.ch
www.karger.com

0304–324X/04/0501–0035$21.00/0

Accessible online at:
www.karger.com/ger

Marja Aartsen
Department of Sociology and Social Gerontology, Vrije Universiteit
de Boelelaan 1081c
1081 HV Amsterdam (The Netherlands)
Tel. +31 20 4446845, Fax +31 20 4446810, E-Mail mj.aartsen.emgo@med.vu.nl

age and gender, men show less decline in speed and reasoning than women [6].

However, to evaluate intraindividual variability in cognitive functioning and whether men and women differ in rate of change, longitudinal data are needed. There are a few studies that focused on gender differences in rate of change, but results are inconclusive. Larrabee and Crook [8] observed that women showed less rapid decline in delayed recall than men, whereas Finkel et al. [9] did not observe gender differences in rate of change.

The main aim of the present longitudinal study is to evaluate inter- and intraindividual variability in fluid intelligence. More precisely, we describe differences in level of fluid intelligence between men and women specified for immediate and delayed recall, information processing speed and non-verbal reasoning, and whether men and women differ in rate of decline during the study period. We control for level of education as men, on average, are higher educated than women. Although the level of education is an important predictor of crystallized intelligence, due to the interrelationship with fluid intelligence [2] it may also affect fluid intelligence.

Method

Sample

Data are derived from the Longitudinal Aging Study Amsterdam (LASA), which is an ongoing longitudinal, multidisciplinary research project focusing on autonomy and well-being in the ageing population [10]. The general design, measures, and procedures of LASA have been described elsewhere [10, 11]. For the present study we selected respondents who were at least 60 years old at baseline, as the youngest birth cohort (i.e., aged between 55 and 59) was excluded for the assessment of memory and speed at follow-up. We further excluded respondents who might have been suffering from dementia at baseline (23 or lower on the MMSE). Although it can be argued that people at risk of dementia are an integral part of ageing as a population process [7], we decided to exclude them because of the differences in rate of cognitive decline between demented and non-demented individuals [12]. Thus, the study sample consisted of 1,132 men and 1,175 women (74% of total sample) at baseline.

Attrition (n = 755) between T_1 and T_3 was caused by mortality (560 persons, 75%), refusal (115 persons, 15%), frailty (62 persons, 8%), and failure to contact (18 persons, 2%). Attrition is associated with all variables included in the analysis; lower scores on immediate recall (–1.0 word on 15 Words Test) and delayed recall (–1.2 word on 15 Words Test), lower speed (–4 letter-letter combinations per trial of 1 min), lower scores on non-verbal reasoning (–1.7 on a 24-point scale) being male, and high age (5 years older) (all $p < 0.001$) at T_1.

Measures

Cognitive Variables. The cognitive abilities in this study were aspects of fluid intelligence, i.e., immediate recall, delayed recall, non-verbal reasoning and information processing speed. The 15-Words Test [13], derived from the Auditory Verbal Learning Test [14], was chosen for the assessment of immediate and delayed recall. Raven's Coloured Progressive Matrices [15] was used to measure non-verbal reasoning. An adaptation of the Coding Task [unpubl. data] was used to assess information processing speed.

Confounding Variables. Level of education was assessed by asking the respondent for the highest educational course completed, resulting in a variable ranging from 1 (incomplete elementary education) to 9 (university education). Age is presented in years.

Procedure. Latent change models [16] were used to estimate the level and rate of change in the four cognitive functions. With this type of modelling, it is possible to estimate individuals' true levels of cognitive functioning (level), true rates of linear (slope) and non-linear (e.g. quadratic slope) change, as well as the individual variability in test performance separately for men and women. The factor loadings were constrained to be equal across time (factorial invariance). No residual covariances, indicating that errors within or between measurements are correlated, were included. For the one-indicator models (i.e. delayed recall and non-verbal reasoning), we further constrained the error variances of the indicators to be equal across time (homoscedascity) in order to have a positive number of degrees of freedom. When good fitting models were obtained (i.e. CFI >0.95, RMSEA <0.06, SRMR <0.08 [17]), potential predictors of level and change, i.e., age and level of education, were included. The latent change models were estimated with Mplus 2.1 [17].

As a higher dropout rate was related to all study variables (see sample description), missing values in our study sample could not be considered missing completely at random (MCAR). If they were, then a listwise deletion of observations with missingness on any of the variables would not affect the parameter estimates [18]. If observations are missing at random (MAR), which is the case when probabilities of values being missing can be predicted by variables that are not missing [17], then a better approach is to use incomplete data and estimate all missing values based on observation on the variables that are not missing. Mplus performs maximum-likelihood estimation under MAR.

Results

Two estimated parameters are of particular interest, i.e. level and slope, and in the case of non-linear change, quadratic slope [2]. The estimated levels and slopes for the four cognitive abilities are estimated separately for men and women (table 1). The levels describe the true level of cognitive functioning, adjusted for age and level of education. The slopes describe the annual rate of change during the time in study, adjusted for age and level of education.

All models fitted the data moderately (delayed recall) to excellent (non-verbal reasoning). The 95% confidence intervals (CIs) indicate whether the parameters significantly differ from zero (zero not included in the CIs), or whether parameters differ significantly from each other (no overlap in CIs). According to the levels and the accompanying CIs, it appeared that women had higher levels of immediate recall (+0.50) and delayed recall than

Table 1. Latent level and slope of immediate recall, delayed recall, information processing speed, and non-verbal reasoning adjusted for age and level of education, by gender

Cognitive ability		Parameter	Men	95% CI		Women	95% CI		Fit statistics				
				LL	UL		LL	UL	χ^2	d.f.	CFI	RMSEA	SRMR
Immediate recall	M	level	***4.09***	4.01	4.20	***4.59***	4.52	4.71	(men)				
		slope	**0.26**	0.18	0.34	**0.23**	0.13	0.29	97.87	34	0.99	0.04	0.04
		slope^2	**−0.20**	−0.25	−0.14	**−0.19**	−0.22	−0.11	(women)				
	Var	level	**1.32**	1.07	1.56	**1.36**	1.10	1.61	89.90	34	0.99	0.04	0.04
		slope	**0.02**	0.01	0.03	0.01	0.00	0.02					
Delayed recall	M	level	***4.28***	4.15	4.46	***5.53***	5.40	5.74	(men)				
		slope	**0.59**	0.42	0.74	**0.74**	0.52	0.86	12.46	2	0.98	0.07	0.05
		slope^2	**−0.44**	−0.53	−0.32	**−0.53**	−0.61	−0.39	(women)				
	Var	level	**3.57**	3.01	4.21	**4.53**	3.87	5.34	16.11	2	0.98	0.08	0.07
		slope	0.02	−0.01	0.05	**0.04**	0.01	0.07					
Information processing speed	M	level	**21.74**	21.44	22.26	**22.03**	21.76	22.60	(men)				
		slope	**−0.36**	−0.39	−0.29	**−0.30**	−0.33	−0.24	130.50	35	0.99	0.05	0.03
	Var	level	**38.10**	33.68	42.63	**42.57**	38.57	47.93	(women)				
		slope	0.17	−0.00	0.34	**0.16**	0.06	0.38	125.08	35	0.99	0.05	0.04
Non-verbal reasoning	M	level	**17.95**	17.71	18.18	**17.59**	17.37	17.82	(men)				
		slope	**−0.20**	−0.21	−0.12	**−0.17**	−0.21	−0.13	3.32	3	1.00	0.01	0.01
	Var	level	**11.00**	9.63	12.36	**9.62**	8.27	10.97	(women)				
		slope	0.05	0.00	0.10	0.00	−0.05	0.05	3.64	3	1.00	0.01	0.02

Significant effects appear in bold, significant differences between men and women in bold and italic (n men = 1,132, n women = 1,175). M = Mean; Var = variance; LL= lower level; UL = upper level; d.f. = degrees of freedom; CFI = comparative fit index; RMSEA = root mean square error of approximation; SRMR = standardized root mean square residual.

men (+1.25). Differences between men and women in level of information processing speed and non-verbal reasoning were not significant. The variances of the estimated levels indicate substantial interindividual variability in level of functioning within men and women.

The estimated slopes provide information on the annual rate of change. As quadratic slopes make a visual evaluation rather complicated, we calculated the average total amount of change over 6 years in the four cognitive abilities separately for men and women. There was significant linear and non-linear decline in immediate recall (total decline: –0.24 for men, and –0.33 for women) and delayed recall (total decline: –0.42 for men, and –0.33 for women), and significant linear decline in information processing speed (total decline: –2.16 for men, and –1.80 for women) and non-verbal reasoning (total decline: –1.20 for men, and –1.02 for women). Gender differences in rate of decline did not reach the level of significance for any of the cognitive abilities. The non-significant variances of the slope parameters indicate that the rate of change within men and women was almost the same for all individuals.

Discussion

In the present study we described inter- and intraindividual differences in level and rate of change of fluid intelligence, adjusted for age and level of education. Our study revealed that women had higher scores on immediate recall and substantially higher on delayed recall. No gender differences in information processing speed and nonverbal reasoning were observed. Also the rate of cognitive decline was not significantly different for men and women.

The non-linear decline in immediate and delayed recall may be due to an improvement in functioning at T_2. This improvement is often interpreted as a practice effect. In many tests involving learning practice effects can be observed [19]. Practice effects may have been due to the fact that respondents have remembered the delayed recall test, for which they were unprepared at the first measurement cycle. They may therefore have listened more carefully to the words during the third measurement, which resulted in a better overall score.

The finding that women outperform men with respect to immediate and delayed recall is in line with previous research [5]. In contrast to other studies [6, 7], no gender differences were found in speed and non-verbal reasoning. Based on studies on the structure of the brain [4], stronger declines in fluid abilities for men were to be expected. On the contrary, based on studies on the function of the brain [6], stronger declines for women were to be expected. However, none of the findings on gender differences in cognitive decline could be replicated.

Possible reasons for the differences in study results may relate to the differences in methods. First of all, our study results are based on longitudinal data, whereas for the other studies cross-sectional data were used. Cross-sectional studies confound age changes with cohort differences [20]. Apparently, the earlier born cohorts are in less favourable positions than the later-born cohorts, which explains that older people cross-sectionally have lower scores on cognitive tests than younger people. With longitudinal data it is possible to unravel age from cohort effects. Second, with latent change models it is possible to distinguish true change from observed change, by taking into account the effect of measurement errors. When measurement errors are present, it is possible that part of the observed change must be attributed to measurement error rather than to true change. Finally, in the latent change models missing values were replaced by estimates based on the remaining observations, which may reduce the biasing influence of attrition.

To conclude, our study revealed that, on average, the level of fluid intelligence decreases at age 60 and over. We further revealed that women had higher levels on immediate and delayed recall than men, and that there are rather substantial individual differences in level of functioning. Furthermore, in spite of evidence for a stronger age-related atrophy of the brain structure of men, no gender differences in decline of cognitive functions could be observed and interindividual differences in rate of cognitive change are small.

Acknowledgements

This study was based on data collected in the context of the Longitudinal Aging Study Amsterdam, funded largely by the Netherlands Ministry of Health, Welfare and Sports.

References

1 McArdle JJ, Ferrer-Caja E, Hamagami F, Woodcock RM: Comparative longitudinal structural analyses of the growth and decline of multiple intellectual abilities over the life span. Dev Psychol 2002;38:115–142.
2 Horn JL, Cattell RB: Age differences in fluid and crystallized intelligence. Acta Psychol 1969;26:107–129.
3 Christensen H, Mackinnon AJ, Korten AE, Jorm AF, Henderson AS, Jacomb B, Rodgers B: An analysis of diversity in cognitive performance of elderly community dwellers: Individual differences in change scores as a function of age. Psychol Aging 1999;14:365–379.
4 Gur RC, Mozley PD, Resnick SM, Gottlieb GL, Kohn M, Zimmerman R, Herman G, Atlas S, Grossman R, Berretta D, Erwin R, Gur RE: Gender differences in age effect on brain atrophy measured by magnetic-resonance-imaging. Proc Natl Acad Sci USA 1991;7: 2845–2849.
5 Zelinski EM, Gilewski MJ, Schaie, KW: Individual differences in cross-sectional and 3-year longitudinal memory performance across the adult life span. Psychol Aging 1993;8:176–186.
6 Meinz EJ, Salthouse TA: Is age kinder to females than to males? Psychonom Bull Rev 1998;5:56–70.
7 Lindenberger U, Baltes PB: Intellectual functioning in old and very old age: Cross-sectional results from the Berlin Aging Study. Psychol Aging 1997;12:410–432.
8 Larrabee GJ, Crook TC: Do men show more rapid age-associated decline in simulated everyday verbal memory than do women? Psychol Aging 1993;8:68–71.
9 Finkel D, Reynolds CA, McArdle JJ, Gatz M, Pedersen N: Latent growth curve analyses of accelerating decline in cognitive abilities in late adulthood. Dev Psychol 2003;39:535–550.
10 Deeg DJH, Knipscheer CPM, Van Tilburg W: Autonomy and Well-Being in the Aging Population: Concepts and Design of the Longitudinal Aging Study Amsterdam. Bunnik, Netherlands Institute for Gerontology, 1993.
11 Aartsen MJ, Smits CHM, Van Tilburg TG, Knipscheer CPM, Deeg DJH: Activity in older adults: Cause or consequence of cognitive functioning? A longitudinal study on everyday activities and cognitive performance in older adults. J Gerontol 2002;57B:153–162.
12 Reynolds CA, Gatz M, Pedersen NL: Individual variation for cognitive decline: Quantitative methods for describing patterns of change. Psychol Aging 2002;17:271–287.
13 Saan RJ, Deelman BG: Nieuwe 15-woorden test A en B (15WTA en 15WTB) [new version of 15 words test (15WTA and 15WTB)]; in Bauma A, Mulder J, Lindeboom J (eds): Neuro-psychologische diagnostiek. Handboek. [Neuro-psychological diagnostics. Handbook]. Amsterdam, Swets & Zeitlinger, 1986, pp 13–28.
14 Rey A: L'examen clinique en psychologie [The clinical examination in psychology]. Paris, Presse Universitaire de France, 1964.
15 Raven J, Raven JC, Court JH: Raven Manual: Selection 1. General Overview. Oxford, Psychologist Press, 1995.
16 Willett JB, Sayer AG: Using covariance structure analysis to detect correlates and predictors of individual change over time. Psychol Bull 1994;116:363–381.
17 Muthén B, Muthén L: Mplus (Version 2.1) [Computer software], 2001.
18 Enders CK: A primer on maximum likelihood algorithms available for use with missing data. Structural Equation Modeling 2001;8:128–141.
19 Lezak MD: Neuropsychological Assessment, ed 3. New York, Oxford University Press, 1995.
20 Schaie KW: A general model for the study of developmental problems. Psychol Bull 1965; 64:92–107.

Gerontology

Gerontology 2004;50:39–43
DOI: 10.1159/000074388

MMSE Cross-Domain Variability Predicts Cognitive Decline in Centenarians

Matthias Kliegel[a] Martin Sliwinski[b]

[a]Institute of Psychology, Department of Gerontopsychology, University of Zurich, Zurich, Switzerland;
[b]Department of Psychology, Syracuse University, Syracuse, N.Y., USA

Key Words
Oldest old · Mini-Mental State Examination · Cross-domain variability · Cognitive decline · Dementia

Abstract
Background: Early detection of dementia is one of the key issues in cognitive gerontology. However, so far the detection of early stages in cognitive decline has been rather unreliable. One central limitation of current assessment strategies is that they rely on information about a person's level of performance obtained from a single assessment. ***Objective:*** In the first part of the present paper, we propose three strategies for overcoming this limitation by using information from several measurement occasions to improve diagnostic reliability. ***Methods:*** In the second part, we present one exemplary empirical analysis of one of these approaches reporting data from the Heidelberg Centenarian Study. ***Results:*** In this sample of very old individuals tested at baseline and at a follow-up 18 months later, the intraindividual cross-domain variability across MMSE subscales [1] at baseline predicted cognitive decline (i.e. change in an external cognitive functioning rating from baseline to follow-up) much better than baseline mean MMSE scores. ***Conclusions:*** In conclusion, we discuss the advantage of performance varibility as a predictor for cognitive decline.

The development of methods for the early detection of dementia has been a central aim of applied gerontological research for many years. The need for accurate methods of early detection has become even more pressing with the aging of the population and the availability of effective treatments for certain types of dementias that may be most efficacious during early disease stages. However, despite development of highly sensitive psychometric measures [2, 3], our ability to identify individuals in the very early stages of dementia (i.e. years before they reach clinical threshold) has been hampered by inherent limitations of current assessment strategies that rely on information about a person's level of performance obtained from a single assessment. A problem with this approach is the difficulty in distinguishing between poor performance due to low premorbid intellectual ability, preclinical dementia, or state-based fluctuations in cognition [4]. Recent research has demonstrated that only half the individuals classified as high-risk for dementia are *consistently* classified on each of several repeated assessments [5]. The purpose of this paper is to consider alternative assessment strategies that rely on the measurement of variability in cognitive performance.

The reliability of a measurement of cognitive performance reflects the joint characteristics of the specific test and the specific individual being tested. For example, a test of free recall might be very reliable if administered to a sample of cognitively intact older adults, but far less reliable in a sample of neurologically impaired elders because

KARGER
Fax + 41 61 306 12 34
E-Mail karger@karger.ch
www.karger.com

0304–324X/04/0501–0039$21.00/0

Accessible online at:
www.karger.com/ger

Matthias Kliegel
Institute of Psychology, Department of Gerontopsychology
University of Zurich, Schaffhauserstrasse 15
CH–8006 Zürich (Switzerland)
Tel. +41 1 635 3431, Fax +41 1 635 3421, E-Mail m.kliegel@psychologie.unizh.ch

the latter's behavior may be intrinsically more variable. Recent research has demonstrated increased cognitive variability in subgroups of individuals with degraded neurological function [6, 7]. Particularly relevant is the study by Hultsch et al. [6] that demonstrated that individuals with mild dementia exhibited twice as much trial-to-trial variability on simple reaction time tasks than nondemented healthy and arthritic controls.

Efforts to detect individuals in the very early stages of dementia are thus complicated by the likelihood that behavior is most variable (and hence, cognitive assessments are most unreliable) in precisely those individuals at greatest risk for dementia. As a consequence, findings that demonstrate that many individual are not consistently classified as Mild Cognitive Impairment (MCI [8]) across multiple testing sessions [5, 9] may reflect two sources of variability: classification error and amplified intraindividual variability. Hence, variable cognitive performance impairments are likely to precede consistent performance impairments in individuals in the very early stages of dementia. We now consider three possible approaches to addressing these difficulties.

The first is to obtain bursts [10] of repeated measurements in order to estimate *performance variability* and then to use this estimate in conjunction with information about *performance level* to augment predictive validity. In the first step of this approach, one would estimate the magnitude of variability for each individual (i.e. obtaining a measure of within-person variability like an intraindividual standard deviation (SD)). In the second step, one would then add this estimate to information about the level of performance for each person in a model that predicts (early stages of) dementia. This approach is supported by recent work from the Victoria Longitudinal Aging study that demonstrates mildly demented individuals show increased variability compared to nondemented and arthritic controls even after statistically controlling for mean differences between groups [6]. This result implies that using an index of performance variability would have incremental validity above and beyond a single index of performance level in discriminating mildly demented individuals from their nondemented peers.

The second approach is to combine information across multiple assessments to maximize the reliability of performance level estimates for individuals. In this approach, which could be easily implemented in clinical assessment procedures, one would measure people more than once and then take the average of the multiple measures. While typically in clinical memory assessments only one measurement of each indicator is obtained [8, 9, 11], multiple measures will increase the reliability by reducing the error variance by a factor of N, where N is the number of measurements. This holds in much the same way that the SD of the sampling distribution of the mean (i.e., standard error of the mean) is smaller than the standard deviation of single scores in the population by a factor of [(SD single score)/$\sqrt{N}$]. As an example, a common strategy for identifying preclinical dementia is to classify individuals scoring more than 1.5 SDs below the mean of age-matched controls as high risk (i.e. MCI [8]). Long-term longitudinal studies of incident dementia [12] suggests that 5 years prior to diagnosis, preclinical individuals score on average 1.5 SDs below the mean of controls. Assuming equal standard deviations in preclinical and nondementia groups, this yields a sensitivity of 50% and a specificity of 93%. If, for example, the average of 6 scores were used instead of a single score and the same –1.5 SD cut score were applied, the sensitivity would increase to approximately 98% by reducing the effect of intraindividual variability.

A third approach accounts for cross-domain variability across several cognitive measures or cognitive sub-domains at one measurement occasion. While the first two approaches are mainly methodologically driven, the cross-domain approach directly utilizes the theoretical assumption that a decrease in neurological integrity not only leads to increasing variability of performance in one specific domain but also to increasing variability across several (cognitive) sub-domains. Recent evidence for this proposal comes from findings reporting greater inconsistency in cognitive and non-cognitive domains in groups characterized by central nervous system dysfunction or poorer cognitive test performance, respectively [13]. In addition, sporadic evidence has been presented that dropping performance in specific subscales of the Mini-Mental State Examination (MMSE [1]) rather than in the overall sum score can predict cognitive changes in preclinical Alzheimer's disease [14]. Taken together, it seems plausible to assume that the variability of performance across several cognitive sub-domains is a better predictor of beginning cognitive decline than consistently high, medium, or low mean level performance as it is most frequently used in (clinical) cognitive assessment.

While all three approaches have to be tested (more) extensively for their 'added value' in early diagnostic cognitive aging research, in the following part of the paper we will present an example of the third of these analytic approaches to demonstrate that it can optimize the detection of cognitive decline. We, therefore, analyze a sample of very old adults utilizing the occurrence of very rapid cognitive changes in this population.

Method

Participants

The Heidelberg Centenarian Study [15] is a population-based study. All inhabitants of a defined geographical region approximately 60 km around Heidelberg, Germany (comprising 172 communities and 2.6 million inhabitants), who were aged 100, were potential participants. According to this dynamic cohort design [16], there were no other inclusion or exclusion criteria. For recruitment, resident registration offices were asked to provide information on inhabitants born in 1901 or earlier. Overall, 156 centenarians or a close person (proxy) were contacted. 91 of them took part in the study. The main reasons for refusal were health-related problems (50%) or no interest in participation (22%). Except in one case, the interviewer visited each centenarian personally in his or her domestic environment. One (confused and aggressive) woman, although encouraged by a relative, could not be persuaded to meet the interviewer. Thus, at baseline, participation rate in this study was 58.3%, indicating that the sample represented 58.3% of the entire defined population. The average age was mean = 100.2 years (SD = 0.41). Detailed analyses of variables describing the sample at baseline are summarized in Rott et al. [15]. In sum, participants were mainly female, had mostly graduated from primary and secondary school, were for the most part widowed and in half the cases lived in residential care. Every second participant's health state was reported to be good. Compared to the entire defined population, a positive selection seems only to be likely with regard to the participants' health state [15]. After 18 months, we conducted a follow-up on the sample. By that time, 49 of the 91 participants had deceased, 6 of the remaining 42 refused further participation. This left 36 centenarians in the follow-up sample, all of whom were examined on the same measures that had been used at baseline.

Instruments and Procedure

The design and methods of the Heidelberg Centenarian Study have been thoroughly detailed elsewhere [15]. Here, we will merely report the instruments that were relevant to the present purpose. Cognitive status, i.e., the amount of cognitive impairment, was examined with two tests. The first one was the MMSE [1]. We applied a shortened version with which we intended to avoid disadvantages due to sensorimotor impairments when examining people aged 100 years or above. According to initial systematic reports on the problems that can arise in psychodiagnostics in very old people, it is conceivable that contradictory data on very old adults' cognitive status may in part be explained by how cognitive impairment is assessed. For example, Holtsberg et al. [17] demonstrated that on MMSE-items requiring reading and writing skills, sensorimotor impaired centenarians were systematically disadvantaged. Hence, we attempted to minimize biases by using only items that had found to be empirically unproblematic regarding such impairments. We shortened the original test version, leaving out items requiring reading or writing skills and thus reducing the maximum score to 21. The items we used were: orientation (10 points max.), immediate free recall of three items (3 points max.), counting backwards (5 points max.), and delayed free recall of three items (3 points max.). This procedure apparently has no effect on test reliability or validity [17].

As a second, broader measure of overall cognitive functioning and its consequences to everyday functioning, we included the Global Deterioration Scale (GDS) [18], a rating scale to be filled out by a trained interviewer. The GDS is a 7-step rating scale made up of detailed clinical descriptions of seven major clinically distinguishable cognitive stages, ranging from no cognitive impairment to very severe cognitive impairment. Content validity of the GDS was demonstrated by Overall, Scott, Rhodes, and Lesser [19], and inter-rater and retest reliability has been demonstrated regularly at over 0.9 [20].

Results

In the following analyses, we will utilize the shortened MMSE-scale(s) as predictor variable(s) assessing a range of four cognitive abilities: orientation, immediate recall, number, and delayed recall. In addition, the Global Deterioration Scale (GDS) serves as the external criterion reflecting overall cognitive status and its consequences in daily life.

Descriptives

MMSE: At baseline, the mean MMSE score was 10.01 (SD: 7.32, range: 0–21). Distinguishing the four subdomains, the mean score for orientation was 5.03 (SD: 3.85, range: 0–10), for immediate recall 1.88 (SD: 1.31, range: 0–3), for number 2.42 (SD: 2.23, range: 0–5), and for delayed recall 0.68 (SD: 1.05, range: 0–3).

GDS: At baseline, the mean GDS score was 3.97 (SD: 2.09, range: 1–7). 22% of the participants were rated as showing no cognitive impairment, 7% very minor, 12% minor, 10% moderate, 21% substantial, 16% severe, and 12% very severe cognitive impairment. At follow-up, these values changed to M = 4.4 (SD: 2.21, range: 1–7). 19% of the remaining participants were now rated as showing no cognitive impairment, 6% very minor, 11% minor, 6% moderate, 6% substantial, 38% severe, and 14% very severe cognitive impairment. Analyzing intraindividual change (GDS T2 – GDS T1), 55% of the participants did not change in their rating, 6% of the centenarians improved their rating by 1 stage, 19% declined by 1 stage, 14% of the participants by 2 stages, 3% by 3 and 3% of the participants declined by 6 stages.

Prediction of Cognitive Decline

The core question of these analyses was: Can we predict the relatively short-term changes in oldest old adults' cognitive functioning as determined by changes in GDS ratings using information on very rudimentary cognitive measures obtained at baseline? In a first step, we analyzed the correlations between the interindividual variability in MMSE sumscore and the four distinct MMSE subdomains and the intraindividual change scores in GDS ratings. However, there were no significant correlations. In a second step we computed a score of intraindividual cross-

Table 1. Hierarchical regression predicting cognitive change

Predictors	Cognitive change (ΔGDS)		
	β	R^2	ΔR^2
Step 1: mean level performance		0.05	0.05
MMSE Sum Score T1	0.12		
Step 2: variability		0.20*	0.15*
MMSE intraindividual cross-domain variability T1	0.39*		

* $p < 0.05$. β values are taken from the model that includes both predictors.

domain variability. For this purpose we z-standardized all four sub-domain scales and then computed an intra-individual standard deviation across all four subdomains. This measure of intra-individual cross-domain variability correlated significantly with change in cognitive performance ($r = 0.51$; $p < 0.01$).

Finally, we computed a hierarchical regression analysis predicting cognitive change in GDS ratings, including the mean MMSE sum score in the first step and the intraindividual cross-domain variability measure in the second step. This allows assessing the predictive power of the intra-individual cross-domain variability measure after controlling for the influence of mean level performance. As summarized in table 1, while MMSE sum mean level performance at baseline does not explain a significant amount of variance in cognitive change ($R^2 = 0.05$; $p = 0.2$), the inclusion of intra-individual cross-domain variability increases the amount of explained variance significantly ($R^2 = 0.15$; $p < 0.05$). Considering both variables simultaneously, only the intra-individual cross-domain variability at baseline remains as a significant predictor of cognitive change in the investigated population of the oldest old.

Discussion

In the present paper we propose three possible approaches of how to utilize intraindividual variability as a predictor for cognitive decline in old age. In addition, we present one exemplary empirical analysis of one of these approaches analyzing data from extremely old adults who display rapid change in cognitive functioning. Following the research question of 'Can we predict short-term changes in oldest old' cognitive functioning using information on very rudimentary basic cognitive measures obtained at baseline?', the answer was 'yes', but only when considering the intraindividual variability in performance across the four sub-domains of the assessed MMSE version. T1 mean level performance in both the sum score as well as the distinct subscales did not correlate with the observed changes in overall cognitive functioning.

There are a number of possible interpretations for this finding. First, performance variability across multiple domains may be a signature of cognitive impairment in older adults and hence provide a more sensitive indicator of impairment than performance level in any single domain or all the domains combined. Second, the variability score we used may not reflect variability per se but rather differential impairment in some or a single domain, and relative intactness in the remaining domains. Although possible, this interpretation seems unlikely, since the correlations of the individual MMSE scores with decline were small and nonsignificant. Third, on a more general level, the obtained measure of intraindividual variation refers to the heterogeneity of cognitive performance within a person and so contains information about the multivariate status of the individual. Thus, considering this information may be useful for both early detection of cognitive decline and more precise (age-related) assessment of cognitive performance. Although the results from the present study are limited with respect to the covered age range, breadth of cognitive assessment, and size of sample, it seems worthwhile to pursue further studies that assess the utility of using intraindividual variability as a marker of cognitive decline as well as an indicator of the multivariate status of a person and investigating the oldest old as a population of rapid changes.

References

1 Folstein MF, Folstein SE, McHugh PR: Mini-Mental-State: A practical method for grading the cognitive state of patients for the clinician. J Psychiatr Res 1975;12:189–198.

2 Buschke H, Sliwinski M, Kuslansky G, Lipton R: Diagnosis of early dementia by the Double Memory Test: Encoding Specificity improves diagnostic sensitivity and specificity. Neurology 1997;48:989–997.

3 Buschke H, Kuslansky G, Katz M, Stewart WF, Sliwinski M, Eckholdt HM, Lipton RB: Screening for dementia with the memory impairment screen (MIS). Neurology 1999;50:231–238.

4 Darby D, Maruff P, Collie A, McStephen M: Mild cognitive impairment can be detected by multiple assessments in a single day. Neurology 2002;59:1042–1046.

5 Collie A, Maruff P, Currie J: Behavioral characterization of mild cognitive impairment. J Clin Exp Neuropsychol 2002;24:720–733.

6 Hultsch DF, MacDonald SWS, Hunter MA, Levy-Bencheton J, Strauss E: Intraindividual variability in cognitive performance in older adults: Comparison of adults with mild dementia, adults with arthritis, and healthy adults. Neuropsychology 2000;14:588–598.

7 Knotek PC, Bayles KA, Kaszniak AW: Response consistency on a semantic memory task in persons with dementia of the Alzheimer type. Brain Language 1990;38:465–475.

8 Petersen RC, Smith GE, Waring SC, Ivnik RJ, Tangalos EG, Kokmen E: Mild cognitive impairment: Clinical characterization and outcome. Arch Neurol 1999;56:303–308.

9 Bischkopf J, Busse A, Angermeyer MC: Mild cognitive impairment: A review of prevalence, incidence and outcome according to current approaches. Acta Psychiatr Scand 2002;106: 403–414.

10 Nesselroade JR: The warp and woof of the developmental fabric; in Downs R, Liben L, Palermo DS (eds): Visions of Aesthetics, the Environment, and Development: The Legacy of Joachim F. Wohwill. Hillsdale, Erlbaum, 1991, pp 213–240.

11 Burns A, Zaudig M: Mild cognitive impairment in older adults. Lancet 2002;360:1963–1965.

12 Sliwinski M, Hofer S, Hall CB, Buschke H, Lipton R: Modeling memory decline in older adults: The importance of preclinical dementia, attrition and chronological age. Psych Aging, in press.

13 Strauss E, MacDonald, SWS, Hunter M, Moll A, Hultsch DF: Intraindividual variability in cognitive performance in three age groups of older adults: Cross-domain links to physical status and self-perceived affect and beliefs. J Int Neuropsychol Soc 2002;8:893–906.

14 Small BJ, Fratiglioni L, Viitanen M, Winblad B, Bäckman L: The course of cognitive impairment in preclinical Alzheimer disease: Three- and 6-year follow-up of a population-based sample. Arch Neurol 2000;57:839–844.

15 Rott C, d'Heureuse V, Kliegel M, Schönemann P, Becker G: The Heidelberg Centenarian Study: Theoretical and methodological foundations of psychosocial research in the oldest old. Z Gerontol Geriatr 2001;34:356–364.

16 Andersen-Ranberg K, Vasegaard L, Jeune B: Dementia is not inevitable: A population-based study of Danish centenarians. J Gerontol Psychol Sci 2001;56B:152–159.

17 Holtsberg PA, Poon LW, Noble CA, Martin P: Mini-mental state exam status of community-dwelling cognitively intact centenarians. Int Psychogeriatr 1995;7:417–427.

18 Reisberg B, Ferris SH, deLeon MJ, Crook T: The Global Deterioration Scale (GDS) for assessment of primary degenerative dementia. Am J Psychiatry 1982;139:1136–1139.

19 Overall J, Scott J, Rhodes H, Lesser J: Empirical scaling of the stages of cognitive decline in senile dementia. J Geriatric Psychiatry Neurol 1990;3:212–220.

20 Reisberg B, et al: Overview of methodologic issues for pharmacologic trials in mild, moderate and severe Alzheimer's disease. Int Psychogeriatr 1996;8:159–193.

Gerontology

Gerontology 2004;50:44–47
DOI: 10.1159/000074389

Intraindividual Variability and Short-Term Change

Commentary

John R. Nesselroade

Department of Psychology, University of Virginia, Charlottesville, Va., USA

Key Words
Intraindividual variability · Aging · Theories of aging · Longitudinal studies · Longitudinal methods

Abstract
Background: Interest in the study of intraindividual variability is growing rapidly. ***Objective:*** The present collection of papers deals with both longer-term, growth and change and shorter-term intraindividual variability. ***Methods:*** The papers emphasize primarily the former within the context of analyzing large, longitudinal data sets. Also discussed are some key methodological matters. ***Results:*** Criteria to help with choosing methods and modeling with missing data are included. ***Conclusions:*** A promising direction is toward developing a more systematic and intensive conception of the meaning and significance of the wide variety of manifestations of intraindividual variability and integrating them into theories of aging.

Past

The term intraindividual variability covers a wide array of phenomena [1–4]. Two referents, in particular, are germane in the context of this special issue. The first has to do with the kinds of changes associated with learning, development, etc., which reflect more or less permanent changes in the organism. The second has to do with more or less reversible changes such as are associated with mood, state, affective response, etc.

Historically, concern with both kinds of intraindividual variability reaches back to the beginnings of formal psychology. Work associated with processes such as learning and development is familiar through the early research of the likes of Ebbinghaus, Wundt, and others of the experimental tradition as well as the early developmentalists such as Baldwin, etc. Less well known, perhaps, is the direct concern a number of early investigators paid to short-term, intraindividual variability. For example, Flugel [5] systematically studied short-term, performance oscillations three-quarters of a century ago. About that same time, [6] identified and researched the concept of 'quotidian variability' and [7] was distinguishing between unreliability of measurement and 'function fluctuation'.

In addition to the contributions of psychology's founding fathers, much of the current interest intraindividual variability is a tribute to the likes of [1, 2, 8–10], and many others who recognized that the individual could not be captured adequately simply by estimating a series of more or less fixed true scores. Rather, there was much going on with the person that could only be represented in terms of intraindividual variability; and that, for many interesting attributes, meant variability over the short

KARGER
Fax + 41 61 306 12 34
E-Mail karger@karger.ch
www.karger.com

0304–324X/04/0501–0044$21.00/0

Accessible online at:
www.karger.com/ger

John R. Nesselroade
University of Virginia, Department of Psychology
102 Gilmer Hall, PO Box 400400
Charlottesville, VA 22904-4400 (USA)
Tel. +1 434 924 0660, Fax +1 434 982 4766, E-Mail jrn8z@virginia.edu

rather than the long term. New approaches to the modeling of short-term, intraindividual variability data are continuing to appear in a rapidly evolving literature [e.g. 11–14].

Essentially concurrent with a rising interest in the study of short-term intraindividual variability, other researchers were more focused on the kind of intraindividual variability represented in conceptions of learning and development. For example, in 1958 Tucker [15] presented his seminal work on modeling learning data that, through a series of key papers was transmogrified into what is now vigorously practiced as latent growth curve modeling [16–20; see also Ghisletta and Lindenberger in this special section].

Present

Interest in both kinds of intraindividual variability modeling described above is thriving. I have been particularly intrigued and enthused by the burgeoning interest in exploring the nature, predictive value, and implications of short-term intraindividual variability and changes. These interests are symptomatic, I believe, of a broader effort to conceptualize key behavioral and behavioral change matters in more dynamical, change-oriented terms rather than the static, equilibrium-oriented terms that have tended to dominate our history [21].

The present collection of papers, although focusing primarily on the analysis of large, longitudinal data sets, reflects concern with both kinds of intraindividual variability. They also throw in a number of methodological 'bonuses' for the reader, including criteria to help with choosing methods and examples of modeling with missing data. The reader will find much to relish of both substantive and methodological interest in this collection of papers. First, he or she will acquire valuable information concerning available longitudinal modeling procedures, including how to decide what course of action to take and having decided, how to proceed. Second, the reader will get better acquainted with some important longitudinal data sets and learn of interesting analysis outcomes. In their introduction to this series, Martin and Hofer give a concise but informative and thoughtful perspective on short-term intraindividual variability that leads in well to the articles that follow.

Ghisletta and Lindenberger concentrate on two general approaches to modeling longitudinal data – Latent Growth Curve Modeling and Multi-Level Modeling. They identify a series of criteria that bear directly on choosing between the two applications and take us through the decision process and subsequent analytical steps using data from the Berlin Aging Study and the Swiss Interdisciplinary Longitudinal Study of the Old-Old. In their presentation they valuably draw explicit distinctions between static and dynamic concepts and illustrate that distinction within the context of the two models, acknowledging that there are other model possibilities.

Zimprich, Hofer, and Aartsen bring both short- and longer-term intraindividual variability into the same framework by modeling hypothesized relationships between initial cognitive performance and cognitive performance over the long term using data from the Longitudinal Aging Study Amsterdam. They explore and illustrate some of the pertinent issues regarding how this fruitful mixing of time scales can be accomplished with existing modeling software. They find that short-term processing speed changes are related to long-term processing changes and remind us of the potential usefulness of using short-term learning performance as a signal of impending cognitive changes. Their ending note that latent growth mixture modeling may be used to identify sub-groups manifesting different change patterns has salient implications for students of development in general.

Neiss and Almeida not only provide interesting and valuable information on self-reported affect and variability in self-reported affect but also give a timely illustration of how behavior genetic analyses of interesting variables coupled with the examination of age differences can be used to test developmental hypotheses in sophisticated ways. Their finding of no evidence for genetic influences on intraindividual variability further strengthens the idea that intraindividual variability can be a sensitive indicator of ongoing person/context transactional processes as have been studied using P-technique and dynamic factor analysis [e.g. 22, 23].

Li, Huxhold, and Schmiedek home in on the integration of concepts of intraindividual variability in relation to both cognitive and sensori-motor functioning and with theories of aging and also with experimental design. By drawing the distinction between adaptive and non-adaptive intraindividual variability, they set the stage for differential prediction and linkages between intraindividual variability and age as well as a variety of outcome measures. They raise the matter of possible mechanisms for linking intraindividual variability and more basic physiological and biological functions while reminding us of the necessary details that need to be dealt with in order to instantiate such relationships.

Aartsen, Martin, and Zimprich report on another aspect of the Longitudinal Aging Study Amsterdam. They tackle some of the inconsistencies in the cognitive aging literature regarding gender differences while extending gender comparisons beyond level of performance to include rates of change. What appear to be significant gender differences in rates of change when analyzed at the level of observed scores turn out not to be when latent difference scores are modeled. The authors ascribe the different outcomes to both the elimination of measurement error and the use of incomplete data records that are possible with the latent change modeling procedures. The findings illustrate, once again, the long-term bedevilment of change scores but, at the same time, provide substantial encouragement for the use of these more sophisticated latent change modeling procedures.

Kliegel and Sliwinski home in on the prediction of cognitive decline in old age and how it can be enhanced with the use of intraindividual variability information using data from the Heidelberg Centenarian Study. The authors identify three ways to take advantage of intraindividual variability in making such predictions and exemplify one of them – using differential performance within-persons/across-tasks to predict decline – in a concrete example. They make the case well that information regarding level should not be the 'be-all and end-all' of prediction despite the dominance it has held over other kinds of measures (e.g. intraindividual variability indicators) for the last century.

Future

In the context of being asked to comment on work of others done on a favorite topic, it is irresistible not to try to look a bit into the future, if only possibly to stimulate some further developments one would like to see but, alas, on which the 'looker' is not finding time to spend. I believe that the many encouraging findings from the collection of studies of intraindividual variability reported here as well as elsewhere [24–28] have clearly 'raised the ante' with regard to how students of aging build and measure their concepts, design their studies, and model their data.

First, the several applications of longitudinal modeling procedures and the accompanying discussions, including criteria for choosing among alternatives, provide valuable information for others who are trying to understand their longitudinal data. The challenge to model one's data as informatively as possible is being posed and suggestions and guidelines for doing so are made explicit. The burden is on the substantively oriented reader to use this information. It falls on the methodologically oriented reader to build on what is presented here, extending, elaborating, and ultimately replacing these procedures with more powerful ones.

Second, consider the finding that intraindividual variability information predicts over and above what can be achieved by predicting from level information alone. Such intraindividual variability-enhanced predictive validity has been reported by others as well [e.g. 24, 29], so it is not an isolated finding. That said, it is only a small step to acknowledge that if considering intraindividual variability information in addition to level improves predictability, it may improve conceptualization and theory as well. The present set of studies further convince me that door is now ajar. It is time to speculate critically about where we ought to be going in light of where we are now and to plot an appropriate course. I believe a promising direction is toward developing a much more systematic and intensive conception of the meaning and significance of the wide variety of manifestations of intraindividual variability of which we have been made aware and integrating them more centrally into theories of aging [e.g. 26, 30].

Acknowledgment

This work was supported by The Institute for Developmental and Health Research Methodology at the University of Virginia and by a grant from the National Institute on Aging (R01 AG18330-2). I am grateful to the Max Planck Institute for Human Development, Berlin, Germany, for its support of my work over the past two decades.

References

1 Cattell RB: Personality and Motivation Structure and Measurement. New York, World, 1957.
2 Fiske DW, Rice L: Intra-individual response variability. Psychol Bull 1955;52:217–250.
3 Hultsch DF, MacDonald SWS, Hunter MA, Levy-Bencheton J, Strauss E: Intraindividual variability in cognitive performance in the elderly: Comparison of adults with mild dementia, adults with arthritis, and healthy adults. Neuropsych 2000;14:588–598.
4 Nesselroade JR: Elaborating the different in differential psychology. Mult Behav Res 2002; 37:543–561.
5 Flugel JC: Practice, fatigue, and oscillation. Br J Psychol 1928;4(mono suppl):1–92.
6 Woodrow H: Quotidian variability. Psychol Rev 1932;39:245–256.
7 Thouless RH: Test unreliability and function fluctuation. Br J Psychol 1936;26:325–343.
8 Bereiter C: Some persisting dilemmas in the measurement of change; in Harris CW (ed): Problems in Measuring Change. Madison, University of Wisconsin Press, 1963, pp 3–20.
9 Cattell RB, Scheier IH: The Meaning and Measurement of Neuroticism and Anxiety. New York, Ronald, 1961.
10 Wessman AE, Ricks DF: Mood and Personality. New York, Holt, Rinehart, & Winston, 1966.
11 Boker SM, Nesselroade JR: A method for modeling the intrinsic dynamics of intraindividual variability: Recovering the parameters of simulated oscillators in multi-wave data. Mult Behav Res 2002;37:127–160.
12 Browne MW, Nesselroade JR: Representing psychological processes with dynamic factor models: Some promising uses and extensions of ARMA time series models; in Maydeu-Olivares A, McArdle JJ (eds): Psychometrics: A Festschrift to Roderick P. McDonald. Mahwah, Erlbaum, in press.
13 McArdle JJ, Hamagami F: Latent difference score structural models for linear dynamic analysis with incomplete longitudinal data; in Collins L, Sayer A (eds): New Methods for the Analysis of Change. Washington, American Psychological Association, 2001, pp 139–175.
14 Molenaar PCM: Dynamic latent variable models in developmental psychology; in von Eye A, Clogg CC (eds): Latent Variables Analysis: Applications for Developmental Research. Thousand Oaks, Sage, 1994, pp 155–180.
15 Tucker LR: Determination of parameters of a functional relation by factor analysis. Psychology 1958;23:19–23.
16 Meredith W, Tisak J: Latent curve analysis. Psych 1991;55:107–122.
17 McArdle JJ, Epstein DB: Latent growth curves within developmental structural equation models. Child Dev 1987;58:110–133.
18 McArdle JJ, Nesselroade JR: Growth curve analysis in developmental research; in Schinka J, Velicer W (eds): Handbook of Psychology: Research Methods in Psychology. New York, Wiley, 2003, vol 2, pp 447–480.
19 Rogosa DR, Brandt D, Zimowski M: A growth curve approach to the measurement of change. Psychol Bull 1982;92:726–748.
20 Tucker LR: Learning theory and multivariate experiment: Illustration by determination of generalized learning curves; in Cattell RB (ed): Handbook of Multivariate Experimental Psychology. Chicago, Rand McNally, 1966, pp 476–501.
21 Gergen KJ: Stability, change, and chance in understanding human development; in Datan N, Reese HW (eds): Life-Span Developmental Psychology. New York, Academic Press, 1977, pp 135–158.
22 Mitteness LS, Nesselroade JR: Attachment in adulthood: Longitudinal investigation of mother-daughter affective interdependencies by p-technique factor analysis. South Psychol 1987; 3:37–44.
23 Ferrer E, Nesselroade JR: Modeling affective processes in dyadic relations via dynamic factor analysis. Emotion, in press.
24 Eizenman DR, Nesselroade JR, Featherman, DL, Rowe JW: Intra-individual variability in perceived control in an elderly sample: The MacArthur Successful Aging Studies. Psychol Aging 1997;12:489–502.
25 Hertzog C, Dixon RA, Hultsch DF: Intraindividual change in text recall of the elderly. Brain Language 1992;42:248–269.
26 Hultsch DF, MacDonald SW: Intraindividual variability in performance as a theoretical window onto cognitive aging; in Dixon RA, Nilsson L-G, Blackman L (eds): New Frontiers in Cognitive Aging. New York, Oxford University Press, in press.
27 Li S-C, Aggen SH, Nesselroade JR, Baltes PB: Short-term fluctuations in elderly people's sensorimotor functioning predict text and spatial memory performance: The MacArthur Successful Aging Studies. Gerontology 2001;47: 100–116.
28 Musher–Eizenman DR, Nesselroade JR, Schmitz B: Perceived control and academic performance: A comparison of high- and low-performing children on within-person change patterns. Int J Behav Dev 2002;26:540–547.
29 Butler AC, Hokanson JE. Flynn HA: A comparison of self-esteem lability and low trait self-esteem as vulnerability factors for depression. J Pers Soc Psychol 1994;66:166–177.
30 Baltes PB: On the incomplete architecture of human ontogeny: Selection, optimization, and compensation as foundation of developmental theory. Am Psychol 1997;52:366–380.

Gerontology

Author Index Vol. 50, No. 1, 2004

Subject Index Vol. 50, No. 1, 2004

KARGER

Fax + 41 61 306 12 34
E-Mail karger@karger.ch
www.karger.com

Accessible online at:
www.karger.com/ger

An indispensable companion for those involved in clinical trials

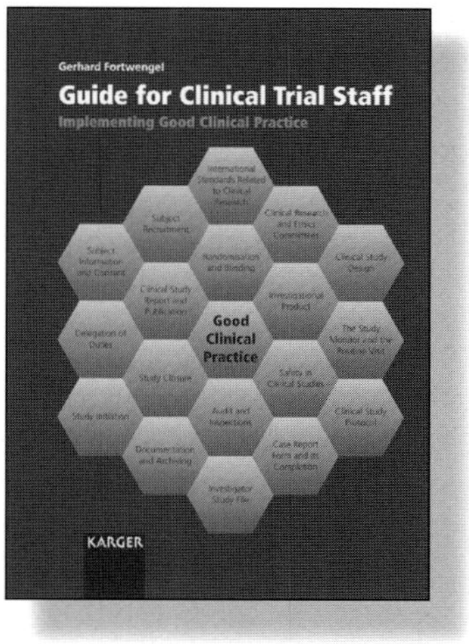

Gerhard Fortwengel

Guide for Clinical Trial Staff

Implementing Good Clinical Practice

General Medicine, Documentation, Communication, Data Processing

Contents

- International Standards Related to Clinical Research
- Clinical Research and Ethics Committees
- Clinical Study Design
- The Study Monitor and the Routine Visit
- Clinical Study Protocol
- Case Report Form and Its Completion
- Investigator Study File
- Documentation and Archiving
- Study Initiation
- Delegation of Duties
- Subject Information and Consent
- Subject Recruitment
- Randomisation and Blinding
- Investigational Product
- Safety in Clinical Studies
- Audit and Inspections
- Study Closure
- Clinical Study Report and Publication

The standard to which clinical trials must conform is called 'Good Clinical Practice' (GCP). GCP is defined as a standard that ensures adequate protection of subjects participating in clinical trials; furthermore, it ensures that all trial activities and data are meticulously documented and reported. The latest GCP guideline was developed by the International Conference on Harmonization (ICH) and was first published in May 1996. This guideline is based on ethical principles that have their origin in the Declaration of Helsinki (1964, last modified in October 2000). Besides GCP, clinical trials must also comply with the local law of the country where the study is being conducted.
This book will be an indispensable companion for those conducting clinical trials and should have a fixed place in the library of every investigator and his staff.

KI 03683

www.karger.com/GCTS

Fortwengel, G. (Basel)
Guide for Clinical Trial Staff
Implementing Good Clinical Practice
VI + 108 p., spiral bound, 2004
CHF 39.– / EUR 28.– / USD 34.00
Prices subject to change
EUR price for Germany, USD price for USA only
ISBN 3-8055-7655-2

KARGER

Order Form

Please send: ____ copy/ies

Postage and handling free with prepayment

Payment:
☐ Check enclosed ☐ Please bill me

Please charge to my credit card
☐ American Express ☐ Diners ☐ Eurocard
☐ MasterCard ☐ Visa

Card No.: ____________________

Exp. date: ____________________

Orders may be placed with any bookshop, subscription agency, directly with the publisher or through a Karger distributor.

Fax: +41 61 306 12 34
S. Karger AG, P.O. Box, CH–4009 Basel (Switzerland)
E-Mail orders@karger.ch, **www.karger.com**

Name/Address: ____________________

Date: ____________________

Signature: ____________________

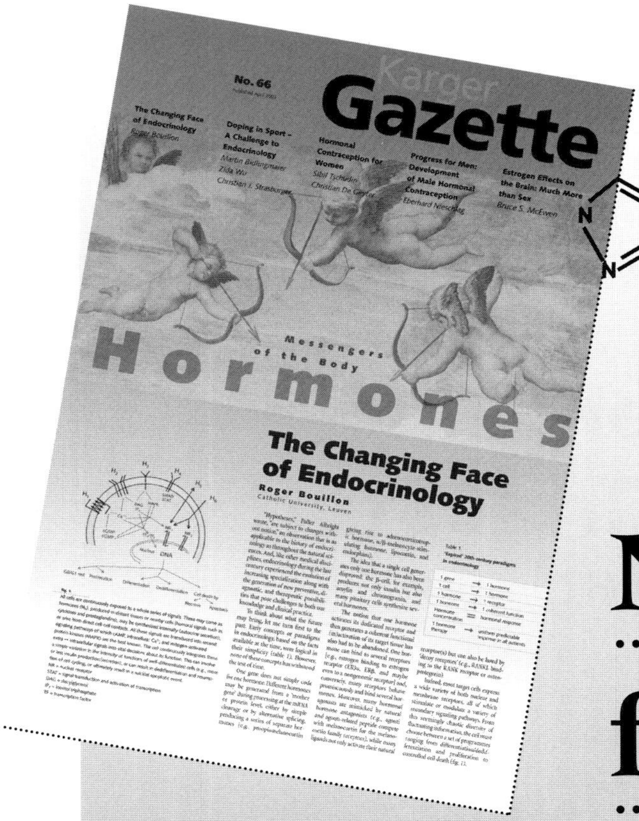

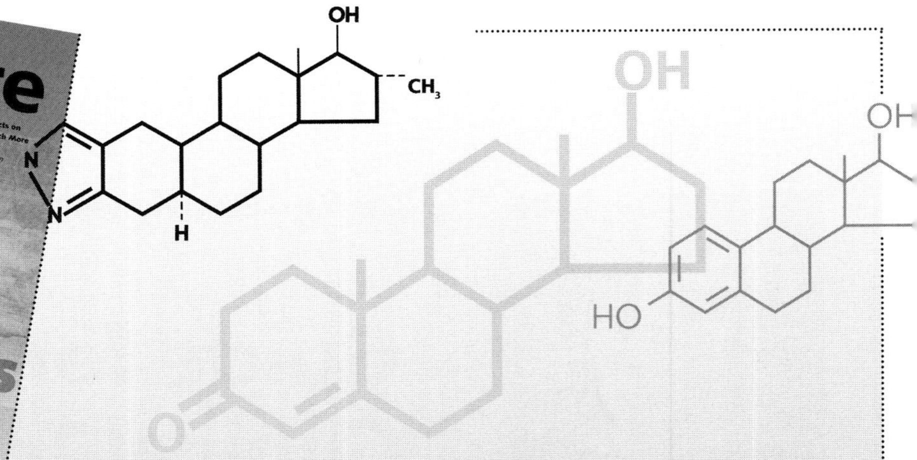

Not just for specialists

The biomedical themes of the *Karger Gazette* are topical, urgent, exciting. Its articles, written by experts from all over the world, provide a wide audience with the basic issues, new findings and controversies in a lively and readable style. Alongside invited contributions, each number carries attractively presented support material, such as informative graphics, historical summaries, interviews, and portraits of individuals and institutions. The *Karger Gazette* appears once a year. And what's more – it's free. To see behind the cover, please write, fax or e-mail us, and we'll start your subscription with the latest issue.

Online: www.karger.com/gazette

S. Karger AG
Karger Gazette
P.O. Box
CH–4009 Basel (Switzerland)
Fax +41 61 306 12 34
E-Mail gazette@karger.ch
www.karger.com

KARGER

☑ Yes, please add my name to your mailing list for my free copy of the **Karger Gazette**

Name: ______________________

Address: ______________________

____

____

____

KI 03254